NEW APPROACHES
TO HEALTH CARE FOR
AN AGING POPULATION

Theodore H. Koff

NEW APPROACHES
TO HEALTH CARE FOR
AN AGING POPULATION

Developing a Continuum
of Chronic Care Services

 Jossey-Bass Publishers

San Francisco • London • 1988

NEW APPROACHES TO HEALTH CARE FOR AN AGING POPULATION
Developing a Continuum of Chronic Care Services
by Theodore H. Koff

Copyright © 1988 by: Jossey-Bass Inc., Publishers
350 Sansome Street
San Francisco, California 94104
&
Jossey-Bass Limited
28 Banner Street
London EC1Y 8QE

Library of Congress Cataloging-in-Publication Data

Koff, Theodore H.
New approaches to health care for an aging
population.

(A Joint publication in the Jossey-Bass health
series and the Jossey-Bass social and behavioral
science series)
Bibliography: p.
Includes index.
1. Aged—Long term care—United States.   I. Title.
I. Series: Jossey-Bass health series.   III. Series:
Jossey-Bass social and behavioral science series.
RA564.8.K63   1988   362.1'6'0973   87-46346
ISBN 1-55542-090-7 (alk. paper)

Manufactured in the United States of America

The paper in this book meets the guidelines for
permanence and durability of the Committee on
Production Guidelines for Book Longevity of the
Council on Library Resources.

Credits are on page 269.

JACKET DESIGN BY WILLI BAUM

FIRST EDITION

Code 8820

A joint publication in
THE JOSSEY-BASS HEALTH SERIES
and
THE JOSSEY-BASS
SOCIAL AND BEHAVIORAL SCIENCE SERIES

CONTENTS

Preface   xi

The Author   xvii

Part One: Providing Services
for the Chronically Ill Elderly

1. The Growing Demand for
   Chronic Care Services   1

2. Responding to the Special Circumstances
   of Chronic Illness   16

3. Chronic Care Services   36

4. Ways of Organizing and Delivering Services   52

5. The Role of the Family   71

ix

Part Two: Developing a Continuum of Chronic Care

6.   Models of Successful Coordinated Care Programs   81

7.   Planning a Coordinated Care System   91

8.   Obtaining Funds   110

9.   Designing Environments for the Elderly   129

10. Implementing a Coordinated Care System   150

Part Three: Administering the Delivery of Chronic Care

11. Essentials of Effective Operation   165

12. Interacting with Chronic Care Constituencies   182

13. Protecting the Personal Rights of the Elderly   196

14. Conclusion: Foundations for the
     Success of Coordinated Care Systems   208

     Appendix A
     Organizations Concerned with
     Aging and Chronic Care   211

     Appendix B
     Summary of Medicare, Medicaid, and
     Private Insurance Coverage for Chronic Care   227

     Appendix C
     Arizona Minimum Assessment Instrument   233

     References   251

     Index   259

PREFACE

THERE IS WIDESPREAD CONCERN among health care professionals about the growing number of elderly people in our society
and the rising cost of providing medical care and supportive
services to those who need them. The inadequacies of Medicare,
changes in family structures, and the devastating effects of age-
related illnesses, such as Alzheimer's disease, are often discussed
but insufficiently addressed in most communities. Adequate
responses to these issues have not yet been developed. In a few
instances, however, pioneering and imaginative programs have
been initiated that point the way to a more humane, respectful, and economically sound approach to meeting the needs of
our aging population. Generally, these programs are referred
to as coordinated systems of care or continuums of care.

Much has been written about the graying of our society,
but very little has been written about the steps that can be taken
by health care providers to establish and operate coordinated
continuums of long-term care. *New Approaches to Health Care for
an Aging Population* has been written to provide a concise descrip-
tion of these steps. This book draws a composite picture of some

of the most innovative programs of chronic care services existant in the United States. My intention in writing this book is to provide a firm foundation of knowledge about chronic care programs for the aged.

My perspective is that of an experienced director who has guided the development of a successful continuum of care program, which is now a significant component of the Pima County Aging and Medical Services in Tucson, Arizona. I discuss this example of a chronic care continuum in detail and also present four other successful models. From these five illustrations I derive practical guidelines that readers can use in establishing a coordinated system of long-term care.

This book is concerned primarily with the development of new approaches to providing services for the chronically ill elderly. It is important to acknowledge, however, that other groups who suffer from chronic disabling illnesses could also benefit from coordinated programs designed to respond to their special needs. Identification of such groups—including people of all ages with physical and developmental disabilities and chronic mental illnesses—is helpful in illustrating the broad scope of the problem. The coordinated systems of care for the elderly described in this book should be equally useful as models for chronic care services for these other groups as well.

Terminology

It is important to recognize that as we examine long-term care many established concepts will need to be modified. New ideas and types of programs will be introduced, existing ideas will be reorganized, and a new language will emerge. One area that will need close examination is the terminology we use to describe the population served by long-term care. Some of the terms currently used to define this population are *retirees, seniors, senior citizens, the elderly, the aged, the frail elderly,* and *the disabled.* Each of these terms has its own connotations and limitations as an accurate descriptor.

My focus in this book is on the care of all people who are subject to life-style limitations caused by chronic illness, regardless of type of illness, age, or other factors. However, in the context of this volume I prefer to identify this population as *the elderly*.

I will also present an argument for referring to long-term care as *chronic care,* because the latter term more accurately conveys the idea that the need for services is defined by the nature of the illness, rather than by its duration.

I avoid using the term *case management,* because I believe *care coordination* better describes the integration of the many services required by chronically ill individuals.

Audience

Because the market for services to the elderly is expanding rapidly, more and more groups in both the public and private sectors are initiating chronic care programs. This book will be especially useful to public officials responsible for making health policy decisions; practicing gerontologists and geriatricians; health care professionals at hospitals, nursing homes, health maintenance organizations, home health care agencies, and congregate housing services; and students planning to enter these emerging fields. Directors and staff members at these settings will find this volume helpful in developing a continuum of services or integrating their existing programs into a coordinated system of long-term care. In order to write a comprehensive manual for these readers, I have addressed the following questions in this volume:

How can I design a long-term-care system within which I can function effectively and economically?

Why can't I organize a long-term-care system in the same way I have structured other services?

What components should an effective continuum of services include?

From what official agencies must I receive approval or licensure?

With what other agencies must I interact in some way?

What are the extent of my local resources: the labor pool, resources for training employees, sources for innovative ideas?

What are the potential pitfalls, critical issues, and policy ramifications of designing a new chronic care system?

How will my services be paid for?

Is there a possibility of making a profit?

Will I have the ability to develop cash reserves?

Where can I find relevant professional literature?

What professional associations, conferences, and workshops will be helpful to me?

What is the future likely to hold?

Overview of the Contents

In Chapter One, I present a demographic overview of our nation's rapidly expanding aging population. The essential characteristics of long-term care are described in Chapter Two, and in Chapter Three, I examine the components and organizational structures most often associated with chronic care systems. In Chapter Four, I discuss alternative sites for delivery of chronic care, several possible organizational frameworks, and the need for a common terminology among chronic care practitioners. Chapter Five focuses on the family members of the chronically ill who serve in helping roles. Chapter Six describes the five programs I have selected as models to demonstrate how a coordinated system can be developed, become effective, and respond increasingly to community needs. In Chapter Seven, I explain the steps to be taken when planning such a system and, in Chapter Eight, I enumerate implementation strategies. Chapter Nine presents in some detail the special requirements of an appropriately supportive environment for aging people who may be experiencing the diminution of sense perceptions. In Chapter Ten, my major concern is how to finance a chronic care program. I examine the existing sources of funding—including a summary of the limitations of Medicare and Medicaid—and take a look at funding resources that might be tapped by new developers of chronic care systems. The smooth functioning of any chronic care system depends largely on three core components: a single point of entry into the system, which I call *controlled access;* patient assessment; and care coordination. In Chapter Eleven, I explain the importance of each of these.

In Chapter Twelve, I examine the roles of institutional administrators and employees of chronic care services and the special characteristics of chronic care that make it different from acute care. Chapter Thirteen emphasizes the importance of helping chronically ill individuals maintain their personal autonomy and their right to choose. And finally, in Chapter Fourteen, as a dedicated and experienced worker in the field of aging I encourage readers to accept and meet the challenge of providing care for our elderly and chronically ill.

Acknowledgments and Dedication

Few individuals have had my good fortune in being associated with so many competent and compassionate people. I have been surrounded by a caring family, wonderful friends, stimulating colleagues, and receptive students. Those who have assisted in the preparation of the manuscript for this volume are identified here with my sincerest appreciation. They include Robert L. Barba, Kristine M. Bursac, Gwendolen S. Butler, John A. Hackley, Marian Lupu, Lana L. Myers, and Richard W. Park. As well, Barbara P. Sears spent many hours discussing the text and word processing the manuscript.

I offer special thanks to the staff members of the five coordinated care programs I have used as models in the book: Geriatrics Institute, Mount Sinai Campus, Sinai Samaritan Medical Center, Milwaukee, Wis.; On Lok Senior Health Services, San Francisco, Calif.; Pima County Aging and Medical Services, Tucson, Ariz.; St. Vincent's Hospital and Medical Center of New York, N.Y.; and San Francisco Institute on Aging, Mount Zion Hospital and Medical Center, San Francisco, Calif.

I also wish to thank the many professional colleagues who contributed to the development of these chronic care programs.

Finally, I feel very fortunate in having the constant love, understanding, and support of my wife, Nancy. It is to Nancy that I dedicate this book.

Tucson, Arizona
March 1988

Theodore H. Koff

THE AUTHOR

THEODORE H. KOFF is director of the Arizona Long-Term Care
Gerontology Center, director of public sector programs, and
professor of management and policy at the University of Arizona
in Tucson. He received his B.S. degree (1951) in psychology
from City University of New York, City College, his M.S.S.W.
degree (1953) from Columbia University, and his Ed. D. degree
(1971) from the University of Arizona.

Koff is the author of *Hospice: A Caring Community* (1980)
and *Long-Term Care: An Approach to Serving the Frail Elderly* (1982).
He has served as a consultant to many groups in the development of chronic care programs for the elderly, and he has in-
structed students and health care practitioners throughout the
United States about chronic care services.

NEW APPROACHES
TO HEALTH CARE FOR
AN AGING POPULATION

Chapter 1

THE GROWING DEMAND
FOR CHRONIC CARE SERVICES

THE NUMERICAL GROWTH OF OLDER PEOPLE around the world is an extraordinary testimony to the improvement of our lives. Increasing numbers of the elderly are associated with relatively high birth rates 60 or more years ago, reductions in infectious and parasitic diseases, reductions in infant and maternal mortality, and improved nutrition. The elderly are also increasing because of worldwide improvements in public and private health services, education, and income.

The growth of older populations poses a considerable challenge to public policy because our needs change as we age. Rapidly expanding numbers of older people represent a social phenomenon without historical precedent, and one that is bound to alter previously held stereotypes of older persons [Torrey, Kinsella, and Taeuber, 1987, p. 1].

The 1980 census reported that 25,000 persons in the United States were 100 years of age or older. This was the first census to report statistics for this age cohort, giving evidence of the increasing significance of the aging of the population. The average age of the U.S. population was 27.9 in 1970; it was 31.5 in 1985.

The following list of facts about aging, prepared by the American Association of Retired Persons (1985, 1986, 1987),

1

contributes an understanding of the importance of developing new comprehensive health and social programs that will respond to the growing numbers of older people who face the possibility of chronic illness and must be helped to deal with it.

- The older population—persons 65 years of age or older—numbered 29.2 million in 1986. They represented 12.1% of the U.S. population, about one in every eight Americans. The number of older Americans increased by 3.6 million or 14% since 1980, compared with an increase of 5% for the under-65 population.
- Since 1900, the percentage of Americans 65+ has tripled (4.1% in 1900 to 12.1% in 1986), and the number increased over nine times (from 3.1 million to 29.2 million).
- The older population itself is getting older. In 1986 the 65–74 age group (17.3 million) was nearly eight times larger than in 1900 and the 85+ group (2.8 million) was 22 times larger.
- In 1986, persons reaching age 65 had an average life expectancy of an additional 16.9 years (18.6 years for females and 14.8 years for males).
- A child born in 1986 could expect to live 74.9 years, about 28 years longer than a child born in 1900. The major part of this increase occurred because of reduced death rates for children and young adults. Life expectancy at age 65 increased by only 2.4 years between 1900 and 1960, but has increased by 2.6 years since 1960.
- About 2.1 million persons celebrated their 65th birthday in 1986 (5,900 per day). In the same year, about 1.5 million persons 65 or older died, resulting in a net increase of over 630,000 (1,750 per day). . . .
- The older population is expected to continue to grow in the future [see Figure 1]. This growth

will slow somewhat during the 1990s because of the relatively small number of babies born during the Great Depression of the 1930s. The most rapid increase is expected between the years 2010 and 2030, when the "baby boom" generation reaches age 65.

Figure 1. Number of Persons Aged 65 and Older: 1900–2030.

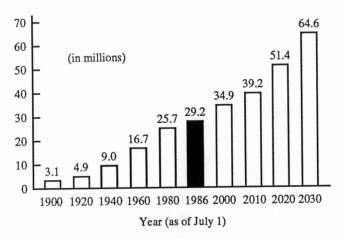

Year (as of July 1)

Note: Increments in years on horizontal scale are uneven.

Source: American Association of Retired Persons, 1987. Copyright (1987). Reprinted with permission of the American Association of Retired Persons.

- By 2030 there will be about 65 million older persons, two and one-half times their number in 1980. If current fertility and immigration levels remain stable, the only age groups to experience significant growth in the next century will be those past 55.
- By the year 2000, persons 65+ are expected to represent 13.0% of the population, and this percentage may climb to 21.2% by 2030 [1986, pp. 1–2; reprinted with permission].

The Social Security Amendments of 1983 initiated a plan whereby the base retirement age, the age at which full retirement benefits are paid, will be increased in 2027 from the current 65 years to 67 years. With increases in the number of persons aged 65 and older, especially those aged 85 and older, the increases in life expectancy, and the recent removal of any mandatory retirement age, society may begin to view the age category of the elderly as beginning at age 70 or older. This would result in an entirely new perspective on expectations for continuing employment and the maintenance of good health. The trend toward the aging of the population is illustrated in Table 1.

Table 1. Trends in Population Aged 65 and Older: 1980–2000.

	Population (by Thousands)			Annual Rate of Change	
Age Group	1980	1990	2000	1980 1990	1990 2000
65–69	8,780.8	10,006.3	9,110.2	1.3%	−0.9%
70–74	6,796.7	8,048.0	8,582.8	1.7	0.6
75–79	4,792.6	6,223.7	7,242.2	2.6	1.5
80–84	2,934.2	4,060.1	4,984.6	3.3	2.0
85+	2,239.7	3,460.9	4,964.6	4.4	4.0
Total	25,544.1	31,799.1	35,036.3	2.2%	1.0%

Source: U.S. Bureau of the Census, 1983.

The 65-and-older population requires more long-term care services than younger groups. Overall demand for long-term care services will increase as the number of people aged 65 and older increases. Table 1 shows that there will be 32 million elderly in 1990 and 35 million in 2000, compared with 25.5 million in 1980.

Although the annual rate of growth in the 65-and-older population is significant, even more rapid growth is expected in the older age categories of this group. The number of persons aged 75 to 84, a key group that uses nursing homes and congregate residential facilities, will increase from 7.7 million to 12.2 million during the next two decades. The number of persons aged 85 and older, the most likely users of skilled nursing and intermediate care facilities, will more than double from

2.2 million in 1980 to 4.9 million in 2000. About one-fifth of this latter group is expected to be in nursing homes at any given time. These trends will place increasing stress on the current supply of nursing home beds.

Some observers point to a number of factors that may diminish the effect of the demographic trends cited previously. For example, it is reasonable to expect that new drugs and technology will continue to make progress in reducing if not deferring the onset of mental and physical disabilities among the elderly. When these disabilities do occur, improvements in the effects of therapy can be expected. Nevertheless, short of techniques to reverse the aging process itself, it is unlikely that technological progress will offset the effect of the increasing number of elderly upon the demand for long-term care (Valiente, 1984).

The Consequences of a Growing Elderly Population

The consequences of a growing elderly population will be noted in more segments of society than that of health care. Increasingly, industry will face requests from employees for time off to care for aged and sometimes frail parents. Personnel benefits have begun to reflect this concern, in recognition that employees have responsibilities for elderly relatives just as they do for children.

When asking employees to relocate to a different community, large corporations may want to identify the resources of a continuum of care for the elderly as an attractive feature of the new area, along with educational and other cultural advantages. Such resources for the elderly may be important to families who face the possibility of aging parents' having to move to a home near their children. Community attractiveness will increasingly be defined in terms of resources to respond to the needs of multigenerational families living separately in the same vicinity. Enterprising personnel recruiters will understand the importance of a chronic care network as a community resource to meet the anticipated needs of the growing population of older people.

In addition, employee health care benefit programs will soon begin to reflect contributions to reserve accounts that will provide for chronic care in retirement. Such provisions should include access to, and payment for, the components of a continuum of chronic care services. Such programs must also take into consideration that many employees will continue to work beyond today's traditional retirement age. Under current health care benefit packages, such employees would be unprotected against the high costs of chronic care.

Community coalitions for chronic care must place the development and support of a continuum of chronic care high on their agendas. For example, because personnel officers are an excellent source of client contacts, sponsors of chronic care systems should establish positive associations with them.

The following data, again compiled by the American Association of Retired Persons (1985, 1986, 1987), underscore the magnitude of the impact an increasingly elderly population must have on institutions and individuals who provide chronic care. (Please note that numbers and percentages followed by an asterisk in the paragraphs and figures below refer to the non-institutionalized population only.)

- The number of days in which usual activities are restricted because of illness or injury increases with age. Older persons averaged 32 such days in 1986 (28 days for males and 35 days for females; 31 days for whites, 43 days for blacks) and spent all or most of 15 of these days in bed (12 days for males, 17 days for females; 14 days for whites, 21 days for blacks) [1987, p. 12].*
- The need for functional assistance also increases sharply with age [see Figure 2]. In 1984 about 6.0 million (23%) older persons living in the community needed the assistance of another person to perform one or more selected personal care or home management activities. This figure represented 20% of noninstitutionalized older persons (17% of males, 22% of females), but the percentage ranged from 14% for persons

65–74 to 26% for persons 75–84 and 48% for persons 85+ . (Selected personal care activities included bathing, dressing, eating, using the toilet, getting in or out of a bed, and getting around inside. Selected home management activities included preparing meals, shopping, doing housework, using a telephone, taking medicine, getting around outside, and managing money. Persons were classified as needing assistance if they needed help from another person or a special aide to do one or more of these activities, or could not do one or more of them at all.)*

Figure 2. Percentage of U.S. Elderly Needing Functional Assistance in 1982.

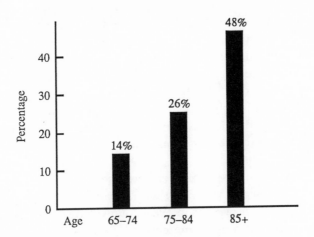

Source: American Association of Retired Persons, 1986. Copyright (1986). Reprinted with permission of the American Association of Retired Persons.

- Most older persons have at least one chronic condition and many have multiple conditions. The most frequently occurring conditions for the elderly in 1986 were arthritis (48%), hypertension (39%), hearing impairments (29%),

heart disease (30%), orthopedic impairments
and sinusitis (17% each), cataracts (14%), diabetes and visual impairments (10% each), and
tinnitus (9%) [1987, p. 13].*

- About 20% of older persons were hospitalized
during 1982, compared with 9% of persons
under 65. Among those hospitalized, the elderly
were more likely than younger persons to have
more than one hospital stay per year (27% vs.
17%) and to stay in the hospital longer (10 days
vs. seven days).

- Older persons also averaged more visits to doctors in 1982 than did persons under 65 (eight
visits vs. five visits) [1985, p. 14].*

- In 1984 the 65+ age group represented 12%
of the U.S. population but was projected to
account for 31% of total personal health care
expenditures. These expenditures were expected
to total $120 billion and to average $4,202 per
year for each older person, more than three
times the $1,300 spent for younger persons.
About $1,000 or one-fourth of the average
expenditure was expected to come from direct
("out-of-pocket") payments by or for older
persons.

- Hospital expenses were projected to account for
the largest share (45%) of health expenditures
for older persons in 1984, followed by physicians
and nursing home care (21% each).

- Benefits from government programs, including Medicare ($59 billion), Medicaid ($15 billion), and others ($7 billion), were projected
to cover about two-thirds (67%) of the health
expenditures of older persons in 1984, compared with only 31% for persons under 65
[1986, p. 14; reprinted with permission].

Figure 3 illustrates the significant increase in the utiliza-

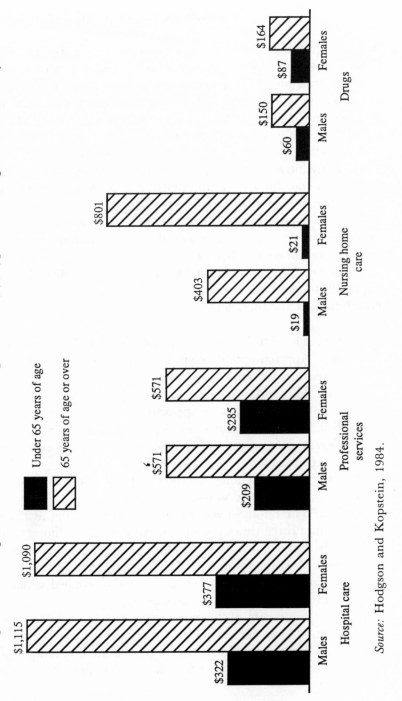

Figure 3. Per-Capita Personal Health Care Expenditures (by Type of Care, Age, and Sex, 1980).

Source: Hodgson and Kopstein, 1984.

tion, by age cohorts, of major health services. Increases in each of the areas of care are startling, especially those related to institutionalization. While increases in the use of each of the services may be anticipated with the aging of the population, it also becomes clear that the most productive efforts to reduce the high cost of services will be those directed toward reduction of hospitalization and nursing home admissions.

Early interventions to promote and maintain good health, as well as coordinated comprehensive approaches to overall health care, are needed to reduce institutionalization, the high cost of this type of service, and the adverse effects of institutionalization upon those who would prefer to remain at home even though beset by chronic illness.

Compelling statistical data support the interdisciplinary approach to conditions requiring rehabilitation in the elderly population. They include:

Fact: The elderly sustain six million fractures each year.

Fact: Approximately two million elderly stroke survivors require rehabilitation each year.

Fact: Three-fourths of all amputations are performed on patients 65 years of age and older.

Fact: The elderly consume 35 percent of all medications.

Fact: 30 percent of the U.S. health care budget is expended on the elderly.

Fact: Life expectancy for today's 65-year-old is approximately twenty years.

Fact: The 85-and-over age group is expanding at more than three times the rate of younger age cohorts; this is the group most in need of rehabilitation services.

Fact: More than four out of five persons aged 65 and older have at least one chronic illness, and multiple disabilities are commonplace in the elderly.

Fact: 26 percent of the elderly live at or near the poverty line ($100 per week).

Fact: There are approximately 16,000 nursing homes nationwide, caring for 1.6 million Americans. Projections to the year 2000 are for 20,000 nursing homes caring for 2.3 million Americans.

Almost 8 percent of acute care hospital patients 65 years of age and older are discharged from hospitals to nursing homes annually. About half of these could go home if appropriate support services were available. In fact, about 200,000 persons per year could avoid nursing home care if they had access to a geriatric evaluation unit (Firshein, 1985).

In 1986 there were thirty-one preadmission screening programs that evaluated nursing home applicants prior to admission. More than two-thirds of these operated on a statewide basis, and most were run by the state Medicaid agency for the purpose of determining Medicaid eligibility. Three states also required mandatory screening for private-pay applicants in an initiative designed to direct the consumer to programs that would be responsive to individuals' needs and thereby reduce personal expenditures for long-term care and postpone the need for public financial support.

Valiente (1984) says that long-term care providers must make a $49 billion capital investment by 1990 and an additional $82 billion investment by 2000 in order to meet the apparent demand for long-term care services until the end of the century. For nursing homes alone, this implies the development of more than one 120-bed facility per day over the next five to ten years. Such an investment will be necessary even if there is a substantial shift to noninstitutional care for many long-term care services.

The issue presented by Valiente is not that a choice must be made between one service (nursing homes) and another (noninstitutional care) but that there is a real need for a comprehensive system that is responsive to the growing number of older people. There are at this time 14,325 skilled and intermediate care nursing facilities among a total of 19,100 nursing homes; these nursing homes provide care for approximately 1.6 million Americans each year at a cost of more than $30 billion (National Center for Health Statistics, 1987). In 1984 there were in the United States approximately 26 million persons aged 65 and older who were living in communities (outside nursing homes or other institutions) (Kovar, 1986). Only a small proportion of these persons had used in-home services; approximately 1 percent had employed homemaker services, and approximately 2 percent had used home health aides. Almost four-fifths of persons aged 65 and older had never used either of these services (Stone, 1986).

Twenty-two percent of elderly persons living in the community had used other community services during 1984, based on Stone's (1986) study of a sample of such persons aged 65 and older. The most frequently used community service was the senior center; approximately 4 million persons aged 65 and older, or 15 percent of the elderly population, reported use of this service in the year preceding the survey. About 8 percent of the survey population also reported having eaten meals at a senior center.

The number and percentage of elderly persons who used one or more community services are shown in Tables 2 and 3.

Table 2. Population Estimates and Percentage of Persons Aged 65 and Older Living in the Community Who Had Used Community Services During the Preceding Year: United States, January–June 1984.

Service	Population (in Thousands)	Use of Services (in Percent)
Total estimated population	26,290	100.0
Senior center	3,970	15.1
Senior center meals	2,057	7.8
Special transportation for the elderly	1,231	4.3
Telephone call check service	*	*
Home-delivered meals	497	1.9
Homemaker service	376	1.4
Visiting nurses	75	2.9
Home health aide	425	1.6
Adult day care	*	*

*Number of responses too small to permit national estimates.

Source: Stone, 1986.

Table 3. Percentage Distribution of Persons Aged 65 and Older Living in the Community by Number of Community Services Used in the Preceding Year: United States, January–June 1984.

Services Used	Population (in Thousands)	Use of Services (in Percent)
Total estimated population	26,290	100.0
0	20,638	78.5
1 or more	5,652	21.5
1 only	2,997	11.4
2 only	1,945	7.4
3 or more	710	2.7

Source: Stone, 1986.

In 1981 national expenditures for all forms of in-home health and social services were estimated to be $3.1 billion, or a little more than 1 percent of total national health expenditures and approximately one-eighth the amount spent on nursing home care (Firman, 1983). As Firman notes, "Barring a series of major biomedical breakthroughs, the number of persons who are chronically ill and functionally dependent is likely to increase dramatically in the future. If disability rates remain constant for various age cohorts, projections suggest that the number of dependent elderly will increase from approximately 4 million in 1980 to 6 million by the year 2000 and 11 million by the year 2040" (p. 67).

The Future of Chronic Care

This summary of data related to the aging population and expectations for its expansion is presented to illustrate the increased needs for long-term care services and to emphasize the importance of establishing new approaches to the delivery of chronic care services that will both respond to the needs of the elderly and be financially affordable. Data vary by year, and the 1990 census will undoubtedly provide new insights. However, the trends and directions are clearly evident, and the emerging comprehensive long-term care systems must be made responsive to this growing market.

The Congressional Clearing House on the Future (1985b) has summarized the trends and their implications as follows:

> America is faced with a growing population of elderly who will increasingly require long-term health care services. These are services which support the chronically ill and disabled, and include home-based, community-based and nursing home care.

Trends

- The elderly population is increasing in size, with citizens over 85 comprising the fastest growing population group in the United States.
- The size of the American family is decreasing. This will mean less family-based support and increasing reliance on outside services for elderly people.
- The elderly are being forced by public policy to spend themselves into poverty. Currently, only Medicaid, a program for impoverished citizens, provides substantial coverage of long-term care. Middle-class citizens faced with immense bills for long-term care must "spend down" their assets to gain eligibility for Medicaid.
- Cost containment initiatives are restricting existing coverage of long-term care. Recent reductions have, for example, included a $443 million cut in home health care financing over the next three years announced by the Secretary of Health and Human Services on July 5, 1985.

Implications

If the above trends are left unaddressed, we may see the following future directions:

- Decline in the range and quality of health care services affordable to middle income elderly.
- Disequilibrium between an increasing demand for long-term care, and a stable or shrinking supply of long-term care service and coverage.
- Increased threat to the financial independence of the elderly as a result of ''spend down'' upon institutionalization.
- Increased reliance upon expensive hospital and nursing home care as people lose access to home- and community-based care.
- Failure of cost containment measures as current cuts cause cost increases in the long run [p. 1].

Chapter 2

RESPONDING TO THE
SPECIAL CIRCUMSTANCES
OF CHRONIC ILLNESS

IN ESSENCE CHRONIC ILLNESS is the challenge of this era to hospital and public health officials and to the medical, nursing, and other professions concerned with sickness and disability. It is America's No. 1 health problem [Mayo, 1956, p. 9].

For many years, and for many people in health care today, long-term care has meant nursing home care. That definition is no longer valid. Although we may not yet be able to boast of a coordinated system of long-term care in most communities, we have advanced considerably since 1965, when the Older Americans Act and Medicare and Medicaid laws were passed, providing the stimulus for development of a coordinated system of chronic care.

Not just nursing homes but home health agencies, retirement communities, congregate housing, senior centers, and even hospitals are part of long-term care. Obviously, long-term care services must include members of the family as well as the recipient of direct services.

Defining Long-Term Care

According to the Department of Health and Human Services, "long-term care consists of those services designed to provide diagnostic, preventive, therapeutic, rehabilitative, supportive and maintenance services for individuals who have chronic physical and/or mental impairments in a variety of institutional and noninstitutional health settings, including the home, with the goal of promoting the optimum of physical, social and psychological functioning" (Koff, 1982, p. 3).

This definition emphasizes several important characteristics of long-term care.

- First, it refers to *chronicity,* which characterizes most of the ailments of older people; the impairments cannot be "cured." Therefore, the *services must be sustained,* not simply provided for a limited time and withdrawn.
- Second, it refers to *physical, social, and psychological functioning.* These three areas are interlocked and interact; therefore, they cannot be treated in isolation from each other.
- Third, the word *functioning* reflects the view that the way in which the individual functions, rather than the diagnosis alone, determines the nature of the services required.

Elaine Brody added the elements of compassion and entitlement to care in her definition. In her view long-term care is "one or more services provided on a sustained basis to enable individuals whose functional capacities are chronically impaired to be maintained at their maximum level of health and well-being. The underlying values are that all people share certain basic human needs, that they have a right to services designed to meet those needs and to be furnished services when needs cannot be met through their own resources (social, emotional, physical, financial)" (1977, pp. 14–15).

An examination of this definition makes clear how far-reaching and encompassing long-term care actually is.

- It incorporates multiple services, because the needs of a person with a chronic illness generally affect several areas of personal functioning.
- Care must be provided on a sustained basis, because neither the duration of a chronic condition nor the regularity with which intervention may be required can be known in advance. Some services may be needed for only a short time. How long care will be required can be determined only by the individual's needs and functional capacities, however; it cannot be stated as a specific period.

The elements of both the Health and Human Services and the Brody definitions are integral to long-term care and are assumed to be present whenever that term is used in this book.

Other Relevant Terminology

Agreement on standard terminology is likely to be a problem in any emerging field. Because the language of long-term health care is emerging with the growth of ideas, it is evolving and therefore sometimes confusing.

There is an inherent danger in any new field: that of creating new names for existing functions for the sole purpose of demonstrating creativity or uniqueness. The transfer of ideas and concepts—communication—depends upon using *consistent* terminology. Especially when a complex program involving a number of disciplines is in its developmental phase, it is critical that professional personnel, whatever their specialty, agree to a consistent and mutually acceptable taxonomy. Such a taxonomy is still to be developed for long-term care.

The critical need for such a taxonomy is typified by problems associated with the very phrase *long-term care,* which suggests that its governing characteristic is the length of time service will be required. As noted earlier, the existence of a chronic condition and the level of individual impairment are much more significant factors in defining the need for delivery of health care services to an individual who does not require acute, or hospital, care.

Appropriate intervention provided at the right time can result in a reduction, sometimes to a relatively brief period, in the length of time services are required. Thus what we need is a way to designate the nature of care, based on the patient's needs, without regard to the length of time care must be provided. Just as *acute care* is the term used to describe care made necessary by an acute episode of impaired health, health care responsive to chronic illness should most appropriately be called *chronic care*.

The coordinated system of care espoused in this book will henceforth be referred to as a coordinated chronic care system, eliminating the temporal connotation of the "long-term" phraseology.

There is a similar need to establish one term, consistently used, to describe what is now generally referred to as the case management function. While the concept is widely accepted, some practitioners and clients find the term objectionable; they dislike its implication that the "case" (in reality an individual and family) is "managed" by some service agency. This language undermines the dignity of the individual and is contrary to the inherent goal of the proposed system: to enable the client and family to maintain self-sufficiency and competence by retaining responsibility for the management of their own affairs.

For this reason I have adopted the term *care coordination* as an alternative to case management, and I refer to persons providing this service as care coordinators. Here again there is a real need for consensus on the part of care providers to adopt these more sensitive terms as part of the lexicon of chronic care services.

One final inconsistency in chronic care terminology, mentioned in the Preface, is in the terms used to identify the older segment of the population. My preference is to use the term *the elderly* to describe a population that, by reason of age or other factors, is subject to limitations upon its members' life-style as a consequence of chronic illness.

It is to be hoped that chronic care practitioners will soon agree on a vocabulary. In the meantime, the more familiar older terms will continue to be employed in the literature.

The Complexity of Chronic Illness and Chronic Care

It is important to understand the complexity of chronic illness in order to appreciate the complexity of the service system needed to respond to the patient and caregivers, to the illness or multiple illnesses, and to the impact of illness on the individual over some extended period of time. No single or simple approach can be responsive to the multiplicity of needs. It should be evident that the response must be equal to the need—that the complicated presentation of chronic health problems requires effective coordination of diverse services as dictated by the needs of the patient and caregivers.

How chronic illness evolves uniquely for each person and how the person deals with the unfolding of chronic problems is called the trajectory of the illness. The trajectory will vary for each individual and may not be predictable. It need not necessarily represent a decline in the person's functional capacity. The effective intervention of chronic care services should be directed toward avoiding such a decline by building upon the individual's strengths and capacities as well as attempting to minimize the impact of losses and limitations. Obviously, the presence of multiple disease entities will complicate the trajectory, making the projection of outcomes extremely difficult (Lubkin, 1986).

A plan for serving persons who have chronic problems therefore must take into consideration that:

1. *Chronic illnesses are long-term by nature.* Services must be so organized that they provide for repeated interaction over a long time period and are responsive to the complex problems that grow out of a long-term illness.
2. *Chronic illnesses have uncertain prognoses,* resulting in considerable stress for the patient and care providers, and the general course of the illness may be interrupted by episodes requiring acute care. Provision must be made for the patient to move readily from one care level to another.
3. *Chronic diseases require proportionately great efforts at palliation.* Every effort must be made to control pain and discomfort

without interfering with the individual's functional capacities.

4. *Chronic diseases are multiple diseases.* Long-term illnesses tend to multiply, with a single chronic condition often leading to additional problems, making management of the patient's total condition more difficult.

5. *Chronic diseases are disproportionately intrusive on the lives of patients,* causing limitations in activities of daily living and sometimes resulting in social isolation from friends and community activities.

6. *Chronic diseases require a wide variety of services* if they are to be properly addressed by a variety of care providers. The coordination of services becomes an intrinsic responsibility of chronic care.

7. *Chronic illnesses are expensive,* because multiple services must be provided for so long, because institutionalization, when necessary, costs so much, and because of "opportunity costs" to family and friends (Strauss, 1984, pp. 11–15).

Chronic care represents an intervention on behalf of a person who has chronic illness in order to offset the functional losses that result from the illness or injury. The intervention may be introduced to prevent an impairment, to avoid a disability, or to offset the consequences of a handicap. There are multiple options for intervention in terms of the timing of the intervention (at what particular point in the trajectory of the illness does one intervene?) and the intensity of the intervention. Some intervention activities may be advocated even prior to the presence of an anticipated chronic condition in an effort to maintain wellness; such intervention should be considered an appropriate part of chronic care.

Some case illustrations are helpful to illustrate the complexity of chronic care problems and to clarify the multiple resources and approaches essential to creation of a comprehensive chronic care program.

Chronic illness may represent for the patient financial burdens, impairment in capacities for self-functioning, intrusion upon the activities of daily living, ongoing discomfort, and the absence of cure. In chronic illness there is a weakening of the body and its capacities that, rather than being limited to a particular function or predictable period of time, can become pervasive and life-threatening. There may be no expectation of cure, accompanied all too often by an absence of caring, as illustrated in Case Study 1.

Case Study 1: The Importance of Caring—in the Absence of a Cure

Mrs. M. is an 86-year-old female who has suffered from lung cancer and is not mentally capable of personal care. Since the cancer metastasized to her brain, she has been confused, fearful of strangers and of supervision. Mr. M., her husband, is 92 years old and frail, does not drive, and has difficulty conducting all household tasks as well as assisting Mrs. M. with personal care. However, he is highly motivated to keep her at home and feels that it is his "obligation" to care for Mrs. M. and maintain the household. Mr. and Mrs. M. have no family support system, nor are they friendly with their neighbors.

Although the couple's annual income is below the poverty level, it is too large for them to be eligible for the county's community services system, which could provide needed respite and homemaker services; on the other hand, the income is too limited to permit purchase of private care. They are eligible for hospice care, however, to which they have been referred by a hospital because Mrs. M. is in the final stage of cancer and has a life expectancy of less than six months. Hospice care, which the couple has accepted, provides a team approach to caring for the terminally ill in a humane and holistic way.

The hospice team consists of a physician, a nurse, a nurse practitioner, a social worker, and volunteers who are willing to provide homemaking, personal care, and a variety of other services the family may need. The team is available twenty-four hours a day for emergency or respite assistance.

By taking advantage of hospice services, Mrs. M. is able to remain at home, and Mr. M. receives the support he needs without depleting the couple's financial resources.

The complications of chronic health problems can drain the resources of the patient and caregivers and impinge upon the social, cultural, psychological, economic, and spiritual reserves of all who are closely concerned.

Case Study 2 illustrates the complexity of chronic illness, especially when exacerbated by an acute episode or when multiple ailments interact. It demonstrates the importance of searching for appropriate options for care rather than imposing a rigid program on any individual.

Case Study 2: Losing Independence

Mr. L. is a 99-year-old man who has been living alone since he was widowed twenty-eight years ago. He moved to Arizona ten years ago for the warm weather. He has three children, all of whom still live in Arkansas.

Mr. L. walks approximately five miles every day to keep his bowels regular, usually to and from the local university's library, where he reads the newspaper, chats with students, and sits in the sun. He eats two meals a day and prefers a light diet with plenty of vegetables. His home is a studio apartment with few amenities, but he finds it satisfactory because he spends so little time there.

Mr. L. had to be admitted to a hospital after his hip was fractured when he was struck by an automobile in a crosswalk. His hospitalization was complicated by the need for hip surgery, a salmonella infection, pneumonia, and a flare-up of ileitis resulting from lack of exercise.

Discharge planning for Mr. L. was difficult, because he wanted to return to his previous life-style and refused to consider alternatives, such as a board-and-care home or a nursing home. Although he was highly motivated toward walking and participated in physical therapy twice a day, it was believed it would be more than a year before he could ambulate without the support of a walker.

Recognizing Mr. L.'s pride in independence and his uncompromising attitude, the discharge planners called family members in Arkansas for assistance. Because Mr. L. refused to move to Arkansas to live with his children, they chose a local board-and-care home they felt would best suit his life-style preferences. Although unhappy about the prospect, he agreed to try it.

When last visited, Mr. L. appeared to have adjusted well to the home, where he was able to care for his personal needs, spend a good deal of time outside on a porch, and run errands with the caregiver's husband. He said he was happy with his family's decision but looked forward to moving back to his old neighborhood and living alone again.

The presence of chronic problems and the need for chronic care is not restricted to any one age group, although the incidence of chronic illness increases with age. Case Study 3 illustrates the multiplicity of services and agencies required to respond to the complications of chronic illness.

Case Study 3: Chronic Care Is Not Only for the Elderly

Ms. T. is a 35-year-old woman who has cerebral palsy. Over the past two years she had flare-ups of the disease and deteriorated physically. Although she previously could transfer herself with the help of a walker, she became progressively wheelchairbound during that interval and began having difficulty with transfers. She now is unable to transfer by herself and is totally wheelchairbound.

Her case worker felt Ms. T. should be placed in a nursing home because of the amount of daily care she needs, but she refused to enter one. Ms. T. has no family, and the friend with whom she had been living said that that arrangement could not continue because of problems that arose.

Adult Protective Services was involved, because at one time Ms. T. was victimized by a friend, but although physically disabled she is mentally competent and decided to live independently. She rented Section 8 housing, contacted an agency regarding receiving Title XX services, and arranged for personal care three times a week. She receives food stamps, travels by Handicar, and accepts the help of friends and volunteers who come in twice a day to help her in and out of bed.

Ms. T. attends a community college through a vocational rehabilitation program provided by the county, and she participates in support groups. She receives counseling for emotional and adjustment problems through a local independent-living center.

Chronic illnesses may be physical or emotional, or frequently both. References to chronic illnesses in this book do not distinguish between the two but encompass the composite of disorders experienced by the individual and family. For this reason it is essential to recognize that any presentation of services must follow a comprehensive assessment of the individual and of that individual's family supports, including both the limitations and the strengths and opportunities available. Many terms are used to describe limitations associated with chronic illness, and confusion about the meaning of terms may prevent a clear understanding of the appropriateness of a planned intervention.

For example, a person with a functional impairment may be in need of chronic care to prevent further impairment and prolonged interruption of normal activities. This should be viewed as an important part of chronic care, since maintaining constant vigilance to ensure that mental or physical impairment does not take place is more desirable than finding ways to alleviate the adverse impacts an impairment may have on an individual. Early intervention can minimize or prevent an impairment's developing into a disability—that is, something that *dis-ables* ordinary functioning. When any given disability deprives the individual of an *essential* level of functioning, so that the individual requires regular assistance from some other person or resource, that disability has become a handicap. The impairment/disability/handicap relationship can be illustrated as a hierarchy, as shown in Figure 4.

Chronic care services are often able to provide preventive maintenance of an impaired person's independence. The next case study provides some insight into the way a physical impairment can be differentiated from a handicap and illustrates the range of services appropriate to a chronic care program.

Figure 4. Impairment/Disability/Handicap Relationship.

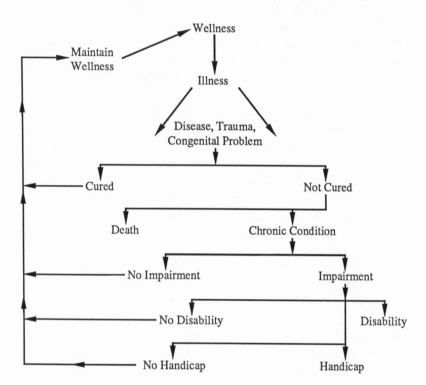

Case Study 4: Determining the Appropriate Service

Mrs. G., an 80-year-old widow living alone, has glaucoma. As a result of her involvement in a community health care program, the glaucoma was detected early through a routine health screening test. Appropriate medication, routinely applied, and regular eye checkups by the health program have resulted in Mrs. G.'s considering the disease only a mild annoyance requiring her to remember to use her drops regularly. The glaucoma is an impairment that was prevented from becoming a disability by the successful intervention of the health care program.

Mrs. G. also has poor vision, an impairment she overcomes through the use of eyeglasses. The availability of large-type books has made it possible for her to continue to enjoy reading her favorite mystery stories. Neither the glaucoma nor poor vision has kept Mrs. G. from working three times a week as a volunteer in a local nursing home, to which she is transported through arrangements made by her health care service.

In preparation for providing services to a person having any chronic impairment, it is essential to determine the extent to which the problem affects the individual's functioning. It is not the presence of the problem that determines the person's needs for service, but the impact of the problem on functional ability. It is only after careful assessment of the impact of the problem on the person's life-style that an appropriate intervention can be selected to strengthen the person's functional capacities and minimize functional deficiencies.

Coordinating Services into a Continuum of Care: A Response to the Complexity of Chronic Illness

A continuum of chronic care services is the purposeful association of health and social services, each having varying elements responsive to the multiple and diverse needs of a chronically ill person and members of that person's family. This clearly differs from a single, free-standing organization that provides services that respond only to a single component of the total array of potential services. For the following reasons a continuum of chronic care is the best structure for organizing the delivery of services to persons who must live with chronic conditions:

- A change in health or competence associated with a particular time of life may not portend a progressive decline. Rather, there may be periods of improvement as well as periods of decline. Any potential for enhanced functioning must be recognized and supported. The availability of a coordinated continuum permits the quick reorientation of services to a more appropriate level of care in response to changing needs.
- The erratic and uncertain nature of the trajectory of chronic illness requires flexibility and resourcefulness on the part of the system. This can best be provided through the coordinated continuum.

- Because chronic illness is a problem for the family and friends of the patient, long-term care services must be available and responsive to changing family involvement in provision of care. This includes providing family caregivers with support, care, and respite. A complex package of services may be needed—and may need to be modified frequently. This flexibility is possible with a continuum.
- Depending upon the changing needs of the patient and the extent of intervention that will be required to maintain or restore function, prevent impairment, or treat illness, there are many chronic care services that could be introduced, and the continuum permits a display of all services and opportunities for choices based on the best fit.
- Funding of chronic care services from public and private resources is complicated by confusing requirements that sometimes result in denial or disruption of needed services. The disruption can be avoided through coordination of the resources of the continuum.

Case Study 5 illustrates the use of the continuum of care.

Case Study 5: Use of the Continuum

Mrs. B. is an 87-year-old victim of Parkinson's disease who has lived alone in her own home since her husband died seven years ago. She was doing very well until she recently fell and broke her hip.

Following hospitalization, Mrs. B. refused nursing home placement and insisted on going home. Her income is well above that qualifying an individual for Title XX community-based services but insufficient to cover the cost of the private nursing care she needs in order to live alone.

Discharge planners were unable to respond to her adamant insistence on returning home and called upon Adult Protective Services (APS) for assistance in resolving her problem. APS called Mrs. B's daughter, with whom she had not been in touch for many years. Until the daughter could arrive to help prepare a longer-term plan, Mrs. B. was transferred to a nursing home.

When she arrived, Mrs. B's daughter learned of the Reverse Mortgage Program, through which an older person can sell a house back to a mortgage holder and receive income from its value. Making arrangements for such a transfer took two months, after which Mrs. B. was able to return to her home.

The daughter had arranged for private home health care on a twenty-four-hour-a-day basis and for a public health nurse to visit weekly.

Although she at first required total assistance in transferring and had some difficulty in feeding herself, Mrs. B. made steady progress. After a year she was able to transfer unaided; after two years, to walk with a walker.

Mrs. B. still needs help with housekeeping, some personal care, meal preparation, shopping, and transportation. These services, which will probably be required for some time, are coordinated by a care coordinator–social worker and they permit Mrs. B. to continue to live at home as she prefers to do.

The concept of organizing all the service elements of chronic care into a coordinated continuum has one purpose: to make it easier for the chronically ill person to have access to whatever services that individual may need. It is not necessary for all the services to be provided through a single organizational structure. Coordination results instead from the ability of all the service components to work together.

There is no requirement that all sponsors have similar structures or funding sources. The critical factors are shared philosophy and goals, a uniform intake and assessment process, and care coordination.

Philosophy and Goal Statement

While each organization within a continuum will have its own philosophy and goals reflecting its uniqueness, the glue that holds the continuum together is a declared statement of mutually shared philosophy and goals related to providing services to people with chronic illnesses. Such a statement serves to guide the development of the planning and implementation of the overall program and provides a sense of cohesion and coherence in these efforts. Further, the statement provides a framework by which to assess the evolution of the program as the needs of the community change and its capacities to provide chronic care grow and develop. The statement of philosophy should recognize:

- That all people are individuals, having different personalities, different values, different interests and avocations, different needs, and different desires and hopes for the future. The chronic care program should respect and support the expression of each person's individuality.
- That the program will be designed to serve persons of all ages, including both those who are chronically ill and those for whom appropriate intervention may prevent disability.
- That it is especially important to provide services that maintain wellness and assist in continuation of a life without the complications of illness.
- That the family and other informal caregivers provide the majority of chronic care services. The program should be designed to acknowledge the vital role of the family in chronic care provision and to help the family sustain this role.
- That chronic care is not merely medical care but a comprehensive response to a person with chronic illness. The programs to be developed and implemented will be integrated and articulated with each other and with the communitywide chronic care system.
- That services will be provided only after completion of an appropriate assessment of each individual's needs.
- That the individual's home is the preferred living and therapeutic environment. Every effort will be made to support the person's ability to remain at home through the provision of in-home services and respite and other support services for family caregivers.
- That at times of severe deterioration of health the person's home may no longer provide the necessary therapeutic environment. The decision to seek institutional services will be made only following a complete assessment of the person's

needs and circumstances and will involve all possible consultation with the person and his or her family. Every effort will be made to support the continuing role of family as caregivers while the person is receiving institutionally based services.

- That the program should endeavor to identify people in need of chronic care services through an active outreach program. Information and outreach should be directed toward enhancing coordination of this program and other community service providers and the development of shared information systems.

The American Health Planning Association (n.d.) promulgated the following goals for chronic care:

The major goal of a long-term care system is to develop a "continuum of care"—that is, a wide range of services and facilities to provide *any* level of care needed by a consumer and to have other levels of care available as they may be needed. A continuum of care includes medical as well as social services, and ranges from total institutional care such as nursing homes and hospitals to less restrictive services or settings such as home health care, nutrition programs, etc. A continuum of care, based on individual consumer need, has a number of objectives including:

- *Rehabilitation*—restoring the individual to some previous level of functioning that can be sustained.
- *Maintenance*—insuring the maximum possible independence of an individual at all times, even if there are limitations on activity or deterioration of functions.
- *Prevention*—slowing of deterioration or anticipating acting on medical and social concerns that are avoidable before they occur.

- *Protection*—providing humane care for persons who are functionally and permanently dependent; assuring death with dignity for those in the dying process.
- *Prolonged longevity*—providing those services that are necessary to maintain life [pp. 8–9].

Each of the five established chronic care systems to be discussed in Chapter Six stresses the goal it outlined in its descriptive literature. Although these goals (included below) have much in common, each is carefully formulated to convey the special concerns of the sponsoring organization and the focus of its services.

On Lok Senior Health Services. "On Lok's goal is to maintain the frail elderly—those over 55 who are eligible for nursing home care—in their own community, and preferably in their homes, as long as it is medically, socially and economically feasible" (*Profile,* n.d.).

St. Vincent's Hospital and Medical Center of New York. "The aims of the program are simple: to help patients remain in their own community, out of institutions, in adequate housing, in the best possible states of health, and at maximum attainable levels of independence" (Young, Harnett, Brickner, and Scharer, 1985, p. 5).

Sinai Samaritan Medical Center. "The goal of the Sinai Samaritan program is 'to help the elderly live independent, healthy, and fulfilling lives'" (*A Step Toward Independence,* 1985).

Pima County Aging and Medical Services. "To develop and offer a comprehensive continuum of care to the community including institutional, alternative, and community-based options in response to community need. To provide appropriate placement within the continuum which maximizes the individual's strengths. To provide supportive services to enhance the ability of the natural support system to provide care in the community. To respond to the needs of all segments of the community requiring assistance with long-term care" (*Case Study,* n.d.).

Mt. Zion Hospital and Medical Center. "We believe that sensible health habits, expert health care, proper in-home assistance, and ample emotional support are the weapons needed to ward off the dependence, isolation, and loss of dignity that often accompany old age. All of the San Francisco Institute on Aging programs share the common goal of helping San Francisco seniors remain independent, avoid institutionalization whenever possible, and enrich the texture of daily life'' (Mt. Zion Hospital and Medical Center, n.d.).

To summarize, then, the ideal chronic care system does the following:

- Has clearly defined goals and objectives
- Emphasizes care in the least restrictive setting
- Maximizes the independence of the person seeking services
- Provides greater incentives for the elderly to remain in their communities and for families to care for them
- Provides a continuum of services that meet the changing needs of elderly populations
- Provides coordinated care (''case management'') and a centralized administrative structure for those seeking services
- Emphasizes services that are community-based and locally controlled
- Is cost-effective in its financing and service delivery mechanisms
- Allows the elderly consumer to maintain his or her dignity and respect
- Allows the elderly consumer to participate actively in all decisions affecting his or her treatment and life-style

Sponsorship and Components
of Coordinated Care Programs

A review of the existing coordinated chronic care programs nationally reveals that they are either part of a public system (for example, a statewide program) or are provided under private auspices with public or private funding supports. This observation is substantiated by Evashwick, Ney, and Siemon (1985), who state: ''Case management has existed in various forms for many years. It has been used for some time by state and local agencies, such as public guardians and departments of public welfare, public health and mental health. Most clients are categorically identified, for example, low income or 'gravely disabled' by mental illness'' (p. 6).

The following table prepared by Evashwick, Ney, and Siemon underscores their point that the history of coordinated systems shows them to have been either publicly supported or demonstration programs.

Table 4. Historical Record of Coordinated Chronic Care Demonstration Programs.

1971: Section 1115 Medicaid Demonstration Projects
1972: Section 222 Medicare Demonstration Projects
1977: Multipurpose Senior Services Project (California)
1978: Nursing Home Without Walls (New York)
1980: "Channeling" Demonstration Projects funded
1981: Section 2176, Omnibus Budget Reconciliation Act (OBRA) Medicaid
1982: Tax Equity & Fiscal Responsibility Act (TEFRA): Medicare contracts with HMOs and CMPs
1984: Robert Wood Johnson Foundation "Hospital Initiatives in Long-Term Care" program establishes twenty-four demonstration projects encompassing hospital-based case management
1985: S/HMO Demonstration Projects implemented (Long Beach, Calif.; Brooklyn, N.Y.; Minneapolis, Minn.; Portland, Oreg.)

Source: Evashwick, Ney, and Siemon, 1985. Reprinted with permission.

It is clear that limited public funding has hampered widespread development of coordinated systems of chronic care. The incentives generally available have been restricted to a specific locale, a specific demonstration, or a special initiative. However, recent changes in health care financing (for example, diagnosis-related groups, or DRGs) have extended interest in coordinated programs to virtually all providers of chronic care, especially those hospitals that receive Medicare funds in payment for their services.

Within the context of this new environment, hospitals have enlarged the scope of their services to include care coordination. This essential component of a comprehensive system may be provided either by the hospital's becoming vertically integrated into a new health system organizational plan or through the purchase of services from a variety of health care providers. In either of these situations, funding will continue to come from public sources, especially Medicare. The issue now has become the survival of health care providers through the creative use of existing funding to create a coordinated system of chronic care.

Hospitals are not the only health care providers that need to explore the possibility of instituting coordinated care services for the elderly. Health maintenance organizations (HMOs) exploring opportunities to enlarge their number of enrollees are understandably reluctant to include new individuals over the age of 65 because of the high costs of providing health care that are associated with more frequent hospitalization and visits to physicians by older persons. But these same HMOs, specialists in managed care, should readily appreciate the opportunities to serve the elderly population while reducing expense through care coordination.

Therefore, health care providers who are either currently serving the population of older people or anticipating entering this service market should become familiar with the content of a coordinated chronic care program as well as the special characteristics of effective management of such a program.

Because the most reasonable approach to becoming responsive to the array of chronic care needs is the development of a comprehensive chronic care system, a fully functioning, well-established chronic care system is recommended as the goal for all communities. In fact, many of the parts of such a system already exist and can be utilized as starting points or can be integrated into an evolving system. Each of the following areas of service represents a critical part of an integrated chronic care system and will later be described in detail: information and referral; controlled access; assessment; care coordination; and provision of services.

Chronic care encompasses services dedicated to the maintenance of wellness and avoidance of chronic illnesses (and the complications engendered by chronic illnesses), responses to family members and other providers of voluntary social supports, payment mechanisms and public policy issues, and the related research activities that are essential to sustain a coordinated chronic care system.

The chapters that follow will describe both the services that are integral to the system and the way in which the entire system can operate.

Chapter 3

CHRONIC CARE SERVICES

THE EVOLUTION OF REHABILITATION for the physically disabled and aged is tied to the growth of social consciousness, with its component sense of responsibility [Lubkin, 1986, p. 354].

Chronic care services are most effective when it is recognized that most people who need them have several problems, not just one. That is why the components of a coordinated system encompass medical, psychological, and social supports and range from occasional assistance to full-time residential care. Giving the individual access to the right combination of services at the proper level at any given time requires the inclusion in a continuum of as many as possible of the following generic services.

Rehabilitation

An overarching characteristic of every chronic care service should be its focus on rehabilitation, or assisting the individual to maintain the fullest physical, mental, and social functioning of which he or she is capable. Rehabilitation in the context of chronic care should also include the goal of assisting the family and social support system to achieve their highest levels of functioning. In other words, the goal is to make it possible for individuals to live as independently as possible in their choice of residence, while continuing their relationships with family and friends.

Rehabilitation is directed to restoring or maintaining wellness or wholeness in the individual and family. It should be employed to assist an individual after some accident, injury, surgery, or illness to maintain functional capacity or to prevent further loss of functional capacity. It is more than merely a medical process, however, especially among the elderly. As Maddox (1987) notes, "Geriatric rehabilitation usually involves a team of professionals that includes occupational and physical therapists and social workers as well as nurses and physicians. The composition of this team reflects the high probability that older adult patients will present multiple health-related problems which have social and behavioral components" (p. 359).

Although rehabilitation is best implemented as a team effort, several professional groups are especially oriented toward this service. Having a physiatrist (a physician specializing in rehabilitation) available to evaluate an individual's needs and to prescribe treatments is of great value. Physical therapy is the rehabilitation specialization most frequently involved and may be joined by occupational therapy, speech and hearing therapy, and therapeutic recreation. In some situations, nurses and nursing assistants with specialized training in rehabilitation contribute to the team approach.

Rehabilitation requires hard work on the part of the client as well as those providing care. It is demanding, and it requires consistent participation and considerable energy. It is often painful. Yet rehabilitation can also be fun, and it is in the context of recreational events that some rehabilitative goals can be implemented through activity programs. In fact, the outcome of the rehabilitation program can be enhanced when it is supported and reinforced through a variety of repeated activities.

For example, the importance of walking for rehabilitation

can be enhanced if the individual participates in a group that regularly completes long walks through a shopping mall. This means of exercising avoids the hazards of traffic and adverse weather and combines the benefits of walking with the added pleasures of chatting with others and window shopping. Obviously there is more incentive to share in this social event than to walk near one's home on neighborhood streets.

As another example, a woman who was alone and depressed after the loss of her husband was helped to join a volunteer hospital group through which she spent several hours each day visiting with children, reading to them, and playing games. She restored her sense of worth and became reoriented to a lifestyle in which she reached out to find new friends among the other volunteers, many of whom also were widows.

The success of any rehabilitation program depends upon the skills of the rehabilitation team, the capacities and motivation of the client, and the expectations of both the professional team and the client that the goals they have set can be achieved. Success can be undermined by the belief that older persons cannot be rehabilitated or that efforts on their behalf are a misuse of professional skills. At the same time, the older person is unlikely to be highly motivated unless the professional believes success can be achieved and communicates that belief.

Any program associated with coordinated chronic care must therefore understand this approach to rehabilitation and be committed to it. As a consequence, expectations and activities that disregard rehabilitation will have to be modified to be responsive to the needs of chronically ill clients. This concern cannot be overemphasized, for it is a fundamental component of comprehensive care.

Counseling

Counseling the elderly, although essentially the same as helping individuals of any age, requires special understanding of the needs of the older person and his or her family, awareness of sources of funds and services, overcoming of stereotypes and negative attitudes about aging, and the ability to relate to the older client as a total and unique human being. Furthermore, services must be seen as offering a significant and meaningful contribution to the life of a person who, although old, has worth. Too often, counseling services are not adequately extended to older people because of their proximity to death and the counselor's own feelings of helplessness in dealing with the ending of life.

Community mental health services generally do not serve many older adults. Counseling is more likely to occur in other settings, such as family counseling agencies, senior centers, nutrition sites, congregate housing, religious institutions, and nursing homes. Counseling agencies and counselors must reach out to the elderly where they are in order to provide the needed counseling services. As counselors provide warmth and human concern for older persons, their skills and talents will help individual clients, those clients' relatives, and clients and families in groups.

Many problems can most effectively be confronted in groups, where participants can benefit from the support and shared experiences of their peers in discussions guided by a counselor.

Another counseling function especially helpful in meeting the needs of older persons can be described as advocacy. In this role, rather than counseling a client, the counselor directs his or her efforts on behalf of the client, calling upon professional insights and skills to enlist the support of others.

The counselor can often assume an advocacy role in environments where the elderly live, receive health care, pursue recreational activities, and spend leisure time, as well as in the many private and public agencies that have an impact upon the lives of the elderly. The counselor may advocate, for example, effective institutional response, appropriate institutional design, and avoidance of architectural barriers.

Counseling for the elderly should be based on the premise that all persons should be treated in the most respectful manner. This includes working to assure that the aging person will not be omitted from the mainstream of our society. Essentially, the most effective counselor role encompasses a successful advocacy position ultimately directed toward full acceptance of the aging person and the absence of need for any special advocacy on behalf of a single client.

Senior Centers

The senior center of today is a community focal point on aging, a place where older persons can meet together, receive services, and participate in activities that will enhance their dignity, support their independence, and encourage their involvement with the community (Leanse, Tiven, and Robb, 1977).

Some senior centers are sponsored by local governments through parks and recreation departments or as components of senior service agencies in the community. Financial support for these may come from local government sources and/or Older Americans Act funds. Other centers are organized as private, not-for-profit organizations that coordinate funding from various private and public sources.

Centers may be located in quarters converted from some other use or specifically built for their purpose. A local Area Agency on Aging can provide a listing of senior centers currently operating in any community. The following list (compiled by Leanse, Tiven, and Robb, 1977) illustrates the wide range of activities that may be found in a senior center program.

Activities and Services for Senior Center Programs

Education	*Information and Referral*
consumer classes	consumer
discussion groups	family problems
health classes	financial
language classes	health
leadership development	housing
lectures	legal
legal classes	nutritional
library services	retirement
nutrition classes	spiritual
writing classes	

Counseling

casework
consumer
financial
health
housing
protective—guardianship
nutritional
retirement
spiritual
legal

Health

clinic
dental
full-time nurse
immunization
part-time nurse
pharmacy
physical exams
physician
screening
therapy
x-ray

Employment

employment counseling
job aptitude testing
job placement
job training

Recreation

arts and crafts
bulletin/newsletter
camping
dancing

movies
music and drama
parties and celebrations
physical fitness
sports
table games
tours, outings, and trips

Social/Community Action

advocacy
legislative testimony
public relations
participation in other
 agencies
speakers' bureau

Volunteering for Center

board participation
committee participation
policy making
teaching classes
clerical

Volunteering in Community

friendly visiting
community fund drives
school aides

Special Services

hearing aid bank
lip reading
special counseling
talking books
therapy (physical, occupational, recreational)
transportation

While a senior center will not usually want to identify itself as a specialized program for older persons who have multiple chronic illnesses, it must be acknowledged that many participants *will* have chronic problems and will benefit from health-oriented programs appropriate to their health status. This reality provides ample opportunities for health care organizations to offer valuable services to the participants at the estimated 5,000+ senior centers now operating nationally.

Persons needing or desiring this level of service may represent between 70 and 80 percent of the population over the age of 65. Since the senior center is undoubtedly the environment in which the largest number of persons can be served at the lowest cost, it is often most appropriately employed to assist persons in the early part of the trajectory of chronic illness.

Case Study 6: Armory Park Senior Center

The Armory Park Senior Center in Tucson, Arizona, is sponsored by the city's Department of Parks and Recreation, with additional funding provided by several grants for specific programs conducted there. Activities of the center are free of charge to all persons aged 50 and older, regardless of income.

An outgrowth of the Senior Citizens Club #1, established under the auspices of the Department of Parks and Recreation in 1959, the center has for ten years occupied a building especially constructed for it—airy, spacious, attractively functional, and completely accessible to the handicapped. As of June 1986 it had served a total of 349,883 individuals in that fiscal year, a clientele made up of 84 percent Anglos, 10 percent Hispanics, 5 percent Blacks, and 1 percent other ethnic groups.

Armory Park Senior Center offers a variety of activities, of which only the federally funded nutrition program is restricted to persons aged 60 and older. Participants may take advantage of field trips, cultural and recreational events, holiday celebrations, arts and crafts, dances, table games, educational and exercise classes, counseling, information and referral services, assistance with applications for benefits (either at the center or at home), transportation, and nutrition education.

Although the city provides major financial support, funds for the nutrition program come through the Pima Council on Aging from Title III of the Older Americans Act. The Kellogg Foundation has earmarked funds for a Nurses' Clinic, staffed by nurses and nurses-in-training at the University of Arizona College of Nursing. The Brookdale Foundation funds a health awareness program called Project Age Well.

Transportation

The provision of transportation is an important element of programs that attempt to help individuals get in contact with their communities and maintain established relationships there. For example, residents of a congregate housing program might regularly attend a senior center activity because transportation is provided by the residential facility, even though it has its own recreational activities. This is an important possibility, since it fosters maintenance of existing friendships and broadens the scope of recreation beyond the environment where the resident lives and dines.

Transportation may be related to scheduled medical care, recreational programs, or church attendance. While most communities provide some limited transportation programs for the elderly, a comprehensive service should provide in its budget for obtaining and operating a vehicle and hiring a driver.

Nutrition Programs

The federal Older Americans Act fostered the development nationally of nutrition and socialization programs for the elderly and continues to provide the major portion of their funding. There were approximately 14,772 such programs functioning in fiscal 1986.

Nutrition centers need not be associated with a comprehensive program, although some of them are located within senior centers that are. The nutrition provided usually consists of a well-balanced hot meal served five days a week. In some settings this is augmented by take-home sandwich meals to be eaten in the evening or on weekends. Some nutrition programs also deliver meals to persons unable to come to the meal site. Home-delivered meals may be made available either on a short-term, interim basis while a participant is temporarily housebound or as an ongoing service to shut-ins.

Nutrition sites may also provide nutrition counseling and other health and recreational programs.

Case Study 7: Pima County Nutrition Sites

Nutrition programs for the elderly were initiated in Pima County, Arizona, by the Tucson Jewish Community Center in 1968 and were funded from then until 1972 primarily through the Jewish Federation of Southern Arizona.

A Model Cities project took over and expanded the program in 1972, and in 1975 a separate entity called Senior Now Generation was funded under Title VII (now Title III) of the Older Americans Act, with funding coming from a direct grant from the Arizona Bureau of Aging (now the DES Aging and Adult Administration). In 1980 Pima Council on Aging was given fiscal and programmatic responsibility for subcontracting nutrition program services.

There are at present fifteen sites at which services are provided at varying levels. These include the city's Armory Park Senior Center, seven Catholic Community Services locations, Handmaker Jewish Geriatric Center, two Tucson Metropolitan Ministries locations, three Salvation Army sites, and the South Park Area Council Center.

Each of the congregate and home-delivered meals provided by these centers provides at least one-third of the Recommended Dietary Allowance for persons aged 60 and older.

Many of the activities associated with a senior center are also offered to participants (socialization, information and referral, health screening, and transportation). Contributions in the form of donations are accepted at all the sites, with suggested amounts at each site determined by a local advisory board. Eleven sites are leased by the Pima Council on Aging for $1 a year; other centers are leased or rented for varying amounts.

Individual providers pay for insurance on the operation of the program. All but one of the sites operate five days a week; the one exception serves meals only three days a week.

Nutrition services are targeted to persons aged 55 and older at all sites. For meals funded by Title III, participants must be aged 60 or older and in social and economic need. United Way support also goes to centers that do not receive SSBG Title XX money. SSBG funds are targeted to persons aged 18 to 59 who are physically disabled but are also available to those aged 60 and older. At the Pascua Indian Center, project income is negligible. At Armory Park Senior Center, where many participants are relatively well off, many pay $1.25 per meal from their own resources.

In fiscal 1987, persons 60 to 74 represented 62 percent of the sites' clientele; 29 percent of participants were aged 75 and older. Only 9 percent were younger than 60. Almost twice as many women as men participated, and the ethnic distribution in 1987 was 66.98 percent Anglo, 22.14 percent Hispanic, 4.39 percent Black, 6 percent Indian, and .49 percent Asian or other.

Home Health Services

The category of home health services encompasses licensed home health care, homemaker services, and personal-care services.

Licensed Home Health Care. Home health care is provided for individuals in their homes for the purpose of promoting, maintaining, or restoring health, or of minimizing the effects of illness and disability and enabling them to live at home as independently as possible. Such service is authorized by a physician and may include nursing; speech, physical, occupational, and rehabilitation therapy; physician services; social work; and counseling. Home health care may be supplemented by homemaker or personal-care services, or the latter two may be provided in the absence of licensed home health care. Medical Personnel Pool, which operates in Pima County, Arizona, provides licensed home health care.

Case Study 8: Medical Personnel Pool

Medical Personnel Pool, which has been providing home care in Tucson since 1973, began working with the Pima County Health Department in 1977. At that time a three-year contract was signed with the agency to provide Title III homemaker–home support services applied for through a case manager. The arrangement resulted in Medical Personnel Pool's developing a caseload of 500 to 600 home care visits per week. The agency was licensed as a home health agency in 1978 and was subsequently certified for Medicare eligibility.

Until 1984, when diagnosis-related groups (DRGs) were instituted, the caseload grew steadily to approximately 30,000 visits a year. Because more patients were being discharged "sooner and sicker" under DRGs, a proliferation of home health agencies was followed by a tightening of rules for Medicare reimbursement, which changed the characteristics of Medical Personnel Pool's clientele. It now provides about 5,000 Medicare-funded and 10,000 third-party-payer intermittent visits a year, plus the equivalent of 208,000 employee hours of typical non-Medicare chronic care service.

Services provided include skilled nursing care (RN and LPN), homemaker and home health aide assistance, rehabilitation services (occupational, physical, and speech therapy), and medical social work. Respite care is an important component of its services, as is high-technology home care required by patients who receive antibiotic IV therapy, chemotherapy, and total parenteral nutrition. A unique program providing cystic fibrosis "tune-ups" helped shorten hospital stays from three to six weeks to three to five days and resulted in great cost savings to chronic sufferers from this disease. Other services are home photo-therapy for infants and early maternity discharge visits to members of HMOs.

A year-long pilot program with Blue Cross/Blue Shield to study the possibilities of supplemental home care insurance (to cover nonskilled services) began in April of 1987 and will employ the case management model, with Blue Cross hiring a case manager and Medical Personnel Pool hiring a home care supervisor.

The majority of patients are 75 to 90 years of age and in the middle- to upper-income brackets, because Arizona's AHCCCS program (its alternative to Medicaid) does not cover home care.

The agency is affiliated with a nationwide concern, Personnel Pool of America (a wholly owned subsidiary of H & R Block).

Homemaker Services. Homemaker services, also known as chore services, are such nonmedical services as cleaning, laundry, meal preparation, and shopping performed for an individual living at home but unable to do these things. Unlike personal-care services, they are limited to services to enhance the physical environment. Personal-care and homemaker services may be provided concurrently and by the same health worker or volunteer.

Personal-Care Services. Personal-care services include nonmedical assistance in such activities of daily living as bathing, dressing, toileting, transferring, eating, and walking. These services are provided to individuals living at home but unable to perform these tasks without assistance. They differ from homemaker or chore services because they directly affect the person rather than the environment.

Adult Day Health Services

Adult day health services can be provided for part of the day in several types of congregate settings to individuals who can benefit from special care but do not require institutionalization. Such services may include health care, physical and/or vocational rehabilitation, meals, personal care, and recreational and educational activities.

A program may be referred to as an adult day hospital service when it is offered within a hospital environment and features intensive health care. Adult day care, a service to the same category of clientele, is more similar to a senior center or recreation program.

Both adult day health and adult day care services may have a specialty orientation; one frequently observed type of program is offered to persons suffering from dementia.

Public financing for adult day health and adult day care programs is limited but may be available through social service block grants or Older Americans Act funds. Some states have requirements for licensing adult day health or adult day care programs.

Case Study 9: Handmaker Jewish Geriatric Center

Handmaker Jewish Geriatric Center in Tucson, Arizona, started its day health care program twenty years ago and now serves approximately 105 persons daily at two facilities. The original center, in space adapted at a nursing home, has generic day health and early dementia programs for persons aged 60 and older. A newer facility, specifically designed to serve its purpose, includes a unit that houses a protective care program for those with Alzheimer's disease and other dementias as well as a program for disabled persons aged 18 to 59.

Each participant in a Handmaker day health care program must receive a social evaluation conducted by a staff social worker and present an updated medical form from his or her physician. On the basis of such evaluation, an individual care plan is devised, including establishment of feasible personal goals. Progress is carefully recorded for each individual, and a semiannual review of the care plan is conducted. A complete evaluation review is completed once a year, with the input of center staff, caregivers, and the case manager or other community-based professional.

Each of the three distinct programs is supervised by a nurse and provides a safe, structured environment appropriate to the condition and abilities of its participants.

The facilities are open five days a week, six hours a day; most participants attend two or three days a week. Of the average total caseload, sixty-five persons take part in the generic program, twenty in the protective (Alzheimer's) unit, and twenty in the disabled adult improvement program.

Both individual and group activities and services are made available, including exercise, personal care, counseling, field trips, shopping trips, meals, socialization, educational classes, reality orientation, and adaptive games. Occupational, physical, and speech therapy are offered on a fee-for-service basis.

Funding for the program comes primarily from Title XX of the Social Security Act, with supplementation from United Way, fees, and donations. Those eligible for Title XX support pay nothing, although donations are encouraged; others are charged according to a sliding scale based on income, with the highest charge set at $26 a day.

Spiritual Supports

Maintenance of a religious affiliation and spiritual beliefs is important to many persons. As people age, the ability to maintain this aspect of their lives is often critical. While attending their familiar house of worship may be difficult because of relocation to a new neighborhood or community, ties to the established spiritual affiliation should be encouraged. This can be accomplished by inviting representatives of religious organizations to institutional settings, providing transportation to a meeting place, or respectfully assisting individuals to follow their own practices.

The Arts

While most institutional programs organize some sort of crafts program, this may not appeal to the cultural interests of elderly individuals whose life-style has included participation in creative activities or attendance at cultural events. Continuing to enjoy these activities is important to those capable of doing so. Obviously, the homebound will not be able to attend cultural events, but their emotional needs may be supported by taking advantage of the broad range of video productions of concerts, dramatic presentations, and other performances that are available.

The Mount Zion program in San Francisco (see Chapter Six) personalizes opportunities to enjoy the arts by inviting local artists to perform for the homebound. When such performers are retirees, this contact often leads to new bonds of friendship based on mutual interests.

Kenneth Koch, an English professor at Columbia University, initiated a poetry writing project in a nursing home, where he worked with a group of persons who had never written poetry. Those who cared for these institutional residents considered them incapable of participating in so intellectual an experience.

To the caregivers' surprise, their patients were stimulated by the expectation that they could think and create and were rewarded by the work they produced. The end result of this project was a book, *I Never Told Anybody: Teaching Poetry Writing in a Nursing Home,* which related the story of their successful venture into the creative arts (Koch, 1977). The program was not viewed as a therapy but as a stimulus to the creative thinking that is part of humanness. It clearly demonstrates the importance of not neglecting the creative aspects of living.

Respite Care

Defined as infrequent and temporary substitute care, or supervision of a disabled person in the absence of the normal caregiver or to provide that caregiver with relief, respite services may be provided through a variety of resources. These include individuals, in-patient facilities, home health agencies, adult day care/health programs, and adult night care.

Respite services are as important to the primary caregiver as to the primary client, but because few formal services include the family or caregivers in their definition of the client, it is difficult to obtain public funds for this service.

Hospice Care

A hospice program provides palliative and supportive care for terminally ill persons and their families. The family is considered the unit of care, and care extends through bereavement. Emphasis is placed on symptom control and pain control for the terminally ill person, support for the patient before death, and support for the family before and after death. Major hospice services include home care, inpatient care, bereavement services, counseling, and education. Medicare law has been amended to include a special hospice provision.

Although, with the possible exception of hospice, none of these services represents an innovation in health care, viewing them as interlocking parts of a system can greatly enhance their effectiveness. The chronically ill person will receive more comprehensive care, the family support system will be reinforced, and the health care resources will be utilized more efficiently.

Chapter 4

WAYS OF ORGANIZING
AND DELIVERING SERVICES

CHOICE AND CHANGE are the two bywords that best characterize long-term care today. In an era marked by declining demand for acute hospital care, long-term care of the chronically ill is beginning to be recognized as a fundamental concern of health care providers [Hughes, 1986, p. 3].

In this chapter I will describe the components that constitute the continuum of chronic care services. A framework within which the array of services should operate, and their organization as a total system, will also be discussed. Because an evolving system is dynamic in nature, the size, scale, and content of services will change in response to the growth of the system, the identified needs of the clients, and changing funding resources.

Designing Services to Meet Client Need

For the developers of a new chronic care system, it is important to note that there are many configurations of services that can respond to the clients' needs. The potential sponsoring organization must explore its own resources as well as those of other community agencies in order to determine what necessary care components are already available, as well as those that are not available and could not readily be made available by a reorganization of existing services. In many cases some of the essential services will already exist in the community and could be integrated into the system by effectively coordinating their delivery to clients of the system.

How chronic care services are conceptualized reflects the sponsoring agency's attitude toward both client and services. Consider, for example, two diverse conceptualizations: a linear and a circular organization of chronic care services.

Figure 5 illustrates a linear representation of a chronic care system. It depicts an approach that is inflexible and does not clearly illustrate appropriate goals for chronic care; it does not make clear that there are individual differences or take into consideration that there may be alternating periods of growth and decline for any individual.

Figure 5. Linear Configuration of Chronic Care Services.

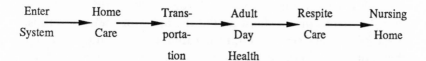

Enter	Home	Trans-	Adult	Respite	Nursing
System	Care	porta-	Day	Care	Home
		tion	Health		

Figure 6, on the other hand, depicts a circular configuration that is client-centered. Through the process of care coordination, the appropriate combination of resources can be invoked on behalf of the client, who is of course a unit including both the primary and secondary service recipients (family and other supportive persons or social resources). This circular arrangement, which illustrates the potential for utilizing a variety of services throughout the trajectory of chronic illness and communicates the reality that both the status of the client and the use of services will frequently change, suggests that the ordering of services is determined by the needs of the client rather than any preconceived hierarchy of services.

Figure 6. Circular Configuration of Chronic Care Services.

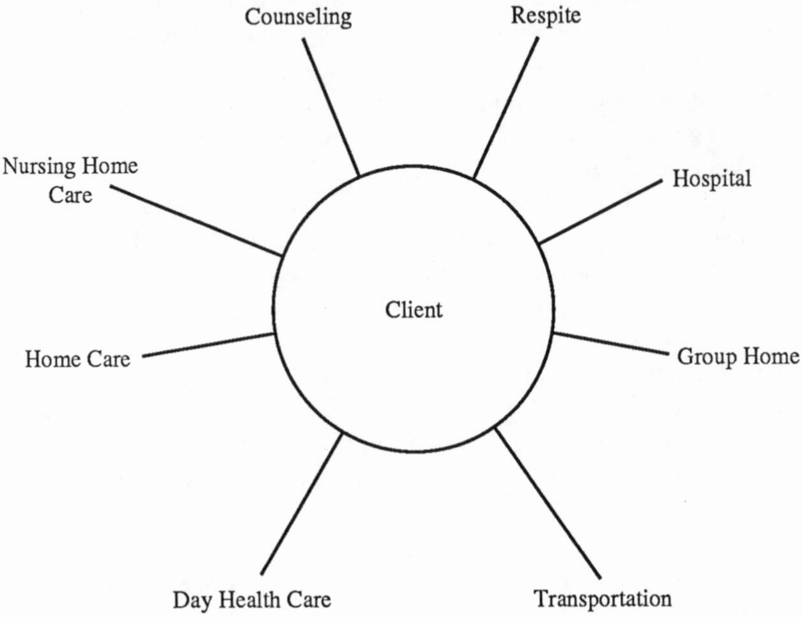

Counseling Respite

Nursing Home
Care   Hospital

Client

Home Care   Group Home

Day Health Care   Transportation

Such a circular depiction forces examination of the individual needs of the client and of the appropriateness to those
needs of the services offered, rather than conforming to a design
that equates a service with a diagnosis. The latter approach
would ignore the importance of an individual assessment that
not only examines the physiological and psychological performance of the client but also explores the manner in which the
client functions in a human interaction environment and how
the social support system has responded to the individual's
changing needs.

Furthermore, because the system organized in this manner is designed to be client-oriented—that is, responsive to the
changing needs of the client—it takes into consideration the place
where the client is when any service is offered. Depending on
the trajectory of the illness, that location may change, thereby
requiring a reconfiguration of the service package. For example, if the primary client moves from the home to a hospital
or nursing home, the secondary client (interested participants)

no longer will be in the same setting as the primary client, and this change may require a different set of responses.

To reiterate, in chronic care:

1. *Services are offered in many locations, not only at home or in nursing homes.* In the trajectory of chronic illness, there may be a need for many different services, some for short periods and some for a long time. It is especially important to distinguish between services provided for those living at home but receiving services elsewhere (for example, at a senior center) and services that are delivered to the individual's home, especially when the individual is homebound.

2. *Services cannot be categorized as "institutional" or "community-based."* Attempting to classify services as "institutional" or "community-based" (home) sets up an artificial dichotomy, because there are multiple levels of institutional care and it is possible to institutionalize at home. If the chronic care system is perceived as a continuum, and if that continuum is viewed as having a circular shape (as shown in Figure 6), then *all* services, including institutions, must be viewed as community-based.

3. *Home-delivered services are always more desirable than institutional services.* While institutionalization in a health care facility is rarely seen as a treatment environment of first choice for treatment of persons having chronic illness, there are occasions when it becomes the preferred treatment. In such instances postponement of institutionalization may impair opportunities for improved health status. However, it must be remembered that the individual's desire to be treated at home should be honored whenever possible.

4. *Home-delivered services may be more costly than institutional services.* Home care services, especially when provided for the homebound who require multiple visits for nursing, physician, or therapeutic services, may be considerably more costly than institutional care, especially when payment for them must be added to the expenses of rent and food. Cost alone should not be the determining factor in arriving at a decision regarding the best site for delivery of services,

however. There may be distinct disadvantages in institutionalization of some individuals, and these should be as carefully weighed as cost.

Possible Models for Chronic Care Services

While services may *generally* be classified as provided either in the home or in an institution, there is in reality a much broader range of options for the location of service delivery. Recognizing this fact expands the alternatives and options for developing chronic care services. To illustrate the importance of making available the most appropriate environment and continuing to stimulate the creative development of new services, four different arrangements, which will be designated models, are presented. These four are not the only possibilities, but they serve to suggest how the scope of services can be enlarged.

1. Community Service Model

In this model clients live at their usual place of residence but receive services at another location—possibly a senior center, an ambulatory care center, or an adult day health center—and then return home each day. Home-delivered services may become part of this model, but on an episodic basis rather than as the primary mode of service. Opportunities for participation in educational, wellness, community service, or other health, religious, or enrichment programs are limited only by the resources of the community and by the individual's access to transportation, scheduling preferences (for example, a preference for daytime rather than evening programs), and interest and stamina.

This model provides opportunities for the early affiliation or enrollment of large numbers of individuals into a coordinated system and emphasizes social and wellness activities.

Case Study 10: Mrs. S.

Mrs. S., a participant in the community service system, lives in the same house where she has resided for the past thirty years. When her husband died, she considered moving but did not do so; she did not know where to go. Instead, she discussed her concerns with the community service agency and learned that she could obtain transportation from a choice of community agencies so that, although she is frail and has limited physical resources, she can spend two days a week at a senior center and participate there in several activities.

She also participates one day a week in a wellness program at a local hospital, which offers exercises, health screening, and discussion groups about nutrition and illness. Mrs. S. is particularly interested in the wellness group, because it gives her access to needed medical care and to pharmacy and home care services. She has been helped to remain at home because of the availability of these community services.

The goal of this model is to stress the availability of a variety of community services that will help maintain the individual's sense of well-being. Participants may provide their own transportation, share rides with other participants or with family members, use public transportation, or be dependent on some special transportation service. While the model does not stress care provided at home, the availability of some additional home-delivered services, such as those required during a period of acute illness, may strengthen this model. Recognition should also be given to the fact that there are many individuals who, although they do very well at home on their own, may occasionally require assistance and rarely, if ever, are seen by any of the community services. Such persons may benefit greatly from being informed of the availability of services and the manner in which they can be obtained when needed.

2. Congregate Housing and Services Model

Congregate housing is a generic term used to describe a variety of housing programs for the elderly that may vary in cost, sponsorship, and number and type of persons served. It consists of housing supplemented with congregate services that may include twenty-four-hour security, transportation, recreation, and meals. These congregate services are what differentiate congregate housing from typical apartment living.

Because of the concentration of large numbers of persons in such an environment, efficiency in service delivery is possible, and residents have the security of knowing they can depend upon having services readily available and getting a quick response from staff in case of an emergency. Modifications to this model include small congregate environments and a variety of types of group homes, although with a smaller number of residents it is less efficient to provide as wide an array of services as can be offered in a large facility, campus, or community.

For the most part, congregate housing programs are located in buildings especially designed for their purpose, although some are in former hotels or schools that have been remodeled and retrofitted for conversion to this type of residence.

Some congregate housing is provided at low rent under public or private auspices. Frequently these units are subsidized by a program of the U.S. Department of Housing and Urban Development (HUD) that makes suitable housing and services available to persons unable to afford a comparable home without such a subsidy. While historically most congregate housing has been provided by private, not-for-profit sponsors, there recently has been considerable growth in development of this type of program by for-profit organizations.

As a result, there are now several ways in which services can be purchased. The first is through a HUD-subsidized program, under either public or private sponsorship, in which the tenant's payments are determined by personal income. The difference between the tenant's payments and the stipulated charges is subsidized by HUD.

In the second type of arrangement, there is no subsidy. The tenant selects a program based on cost, location, reputation of the sponsor, services provided, and space available. A tenant-owner lease agreement defines the responsibilities of each party and, in some locations, an accommodation or entry fee is required. The entry fee may be entirely refundable, amortized over a period of time, or nonrefundable, depending on the lease.

A third arrangement is the continuing care retirement community, or what in the past has been called life care. In this type of housing, for a substantial initial payment plus a monthly fee a commitment is made by the facility to provide housing that includes a variety of types of medical care and sometimes extensive additional health care services, if increasingly required by the tenant. The continuing care concept stresses security for the tenant, who is relieved of anxiety about having to obtain a higher level of care if it should be needed. It is important that the terms of payment be clearly stated in the contract between the tenant and owner, since the arrangement between them encompasses a wide range of services over an indefinite period.

While generally there is a lack of public regulation of congregate housing programs—except for dietary, sanitation, fire, and safety inspections—regulations intended to protect the prospective tenant from fraudulent or mismanaged continuing care programs are emerging through various state insurance commissions. Such regulations require that moneys allocated for future care of the tenant be appropriately safeguarded and available for the tenant's use as needed. There is also a voluntary accreditation program for managers of this type of facility. Developed by the American Association of Homes for the Aging, this program is intended to increase the competence of managers of congregate housing. The advanced age of the tenants, the multiple services offered, and the implied responsibility for the welfare of the tenants all require skillful management and special competence in services for the elderly.

While the primary purpose of congregate housing is to provide *housing*, many programs have affiliated nursing homes offering multiple levels of health care or are associated with home health agencies to provide in-home health care services as needed. Developers often must decide how much health care it will be viable to provide, especially because the availability of health care will make a program more attractive to persons who are older and sicker and less attractive to younger, more independent persons. Another related concern is the phenomenon known as "aging in place." Residents who require more health care services as time goes on often need an increasingly health care-oriented environment. This may be offset by requiring residents to relocate (either to another level of service within the same complex, or elsewhere).

The 1985 annual report of the Lifecare Retirement Center Industry characterizes the typical facility of this type as:

- Owned by a non-profit organization
- Located in an urban area or nearby suburb
- Comprising 200 apartment units and 60 beds for nursing care on the same premises
- Having an entry fee not refundable after 50 months of occupancy
- Including some nursing care in the monthly fee
- Owner-managed without assistance from a management company
- Providing free transportation
- Having been built before 1977 [Laventhal and Horwath, 1985, p. 12]

The congregate housing setting, because of the number of residents living in a single environment, can offer a wide variety of services that it would be difficult to replicate and costly to provide in individual residences or small-group homes. This housing alternative is therefore viewed as an attractive one for older people; it can respond to multiple needs while enhancing opportunities for socialization and a pleasant life-style.

Group homes offer another alternative to independent living. Also known as boarding homes, they provide shared living arrangements for several adults, and tenants may be jointly responsible for food preparation, housekeeping, and recreation. Group homes are not usually licensed and do not provide health care. They appeal to tenants who are relatively self-sufficient but seek some of the services provided by the operator of the home, as well as association with a small number of other persons in an intimate setting.

These forms of housing may be located in a large older home, where the owner leases unused bedrooms and additional space to create a congregate group home. Some older motels have been converted to this type of use, and some new facilities are built specifically for this purpose.

Another variation is *foster care,* in which an individual is taken into a family home with the understanding that a certain level of care will be provided by the foster family.

Case Study 11 describes an example of a congregate living environment that offers comprehensive services to its residents.

Case Study 11: Park Plaza Retirement Residences

Park Plaza is located in the heart of the city of Orange in Orange County, California. Recently opened, it serves a group of older persons who have spent their lifetime in the community, now need additional personal service, but do not wish to move from Orange, where they have friends and familiar places.

This congregate housing facility provides twenty-four-hour security, three meals each day, weekly housekeeping and linen services, recreational activities, and transportation. These amenities reflect the preferences of residents who no longer wish to drive an automobile, shop for groceries and cook, or do heavy housework. No health care services are provided, because this complex is clearly identified as residential, but the reduction of responsibilities and the availability of security, recreation, and full meal service providing balanced nutrition has enhanced the quality of life for tenants.

Although this facility is less than a year old, some of its residents are already experiencing a need for more personal-care services than had been anticipated by the developers. On an interim basis, these needs are being met through a contract with a home health agency, but it is becoming obvious that unless some part of this congregate housing is differentiated as a per-sonal-care area, many of the residents will have to move to a facility that offers the higher level of care that they require.

An interesting approach to calculating the relative cost of congregate housing and continuing to live at a long-time residence is used by Park Plaza and illustrated by Figure 7.

Figure 7. Computing Relative Costs at the Park Plaza.

WHAT DOES IT *Really* COST ?

LIVING AT THE PARK PLAZA COULD COST LESS THAN YOUR PRESENT HOME

COMPARE AND SEE

MONTHLY EXPENSES	YOUR HOME	THE PARK PLAZA
HOUSEHOLD		
PAYMENT / RENT		
UTILITIES		*included*
TAXES / INSURANCE		*included*
WATER, SEWER, TRASH		*included*
GARDENING		*included*
REPAIR/REPLACEMENT		*included*
CLEANING		*included*
TRANSPORTATION AUTO PAYMENTS		*included*
GAS, OIL, MAINTENANCE		*included*
AUTO INSURANCE		*included*
FOOD & HOUSEHOLD SUPPLIES		*included*
LAUNDRY		*included*
SOCIAL / RECREATION		*included*
SECURITY		*included*
TOTAL		

OF COURSE, NO DOLLAR FIGURE CAN BE EQUATED WITH PEACE OF MIND, SECURITY AND A FRIENDLY, CARING ATMOSPHERE. THE PARK PLAZA PROVIDES ALL THE PLEASURES OF YOUR OWN HOME, WITHOUT THE WORRIES.

Source: Park Plaza Retirement Residences, 1987. Reprinted with permission.

3. Home Care Model

In contrast to the community service model, in which the individual lives at home and receives services there, and to the congregate housing model, in which the individual moves to a setting where needed services are accessible, this model shows how services can be provided to the approximately 5 percent of elderly persons who are essentially homebound. This includes persons who may be bedbound.

These individuals require services such as health care provided by physicians, nurses, or social workers, or they receive therapies delivered to them at home. They also may require personal-care services, such as assistance with dressing, grooming, bathing, and eating, and/or homemaking services such as housekeeping and other household chores, shopping, minor home repairs, and adaptations of the home to make the environment more supportive.

Finally, but no less important, they may be greatly assisted by social, cultural, and religious activities that provide stimulation and ongoing identification with the community. Visits by representatives of the church and friendly visitors, or cultural activities such as in-home concerts or craft lessons, are examples of this type of support, expanding the primary provision of this kind of caring by family members.

The model presents many opportunities to explore innovative approaches to enabling individuals to remain at home even when they need significant community services.

Two such innovative approaches, the "nursing home without walls" and the "continuing care community without walls," are currently being demonstrated. Both these alternatives are designed to replicate for persons living at home the supportive services usually provided in an institutional environment or in congregate housing.

As a response to the Lombardi Law in New York State, people who are considered eligible for institutional care can be provided a range of services to enable them to remain at home. This is an important policy innovation, because public funds have generally been more readily available for institutional care than for home care.

The St. Vincent's Hospital and Medical Center of New York home care program, a nursing home without walls program, illustrates how a hospital can use its resources to support people at home. This program offers a combination of home visits by social workers, nurses, physicians, and attendants, with the occasional transportation of the client to the hospital for more intensive ambulatory care services.

A continuing care community that might similarly be designated a "life care community without walls," a concept with great potential, is in the early developmental stage. It would offer participants who pay an up-front fee and a monthly service charge a comprehensive health maintenance package that includes home-delivered services, hospitalization, and nursing home care. The participant would enter into a contractual arrangement much like that involved in admission to a life care facility. The Robert Wood Johnson Foundation is soon to fund several demonstration programs for life care at home, and when the findings from these demonstrations are available, they will add to the existing body of knowledge on HMOs and social HMOs important data on experiences with managed, coordinated chronic care systems.

Whereas the nursing home without walls typically uses public funds that have been made available to assist eligible individuals to remain at home rather than seek institutional care, the life care community without walls would be targeted to a more affluent population. It would serve persons willing to undertake a financial risk in order to be assured maximum protection from the cost of prolonged chronic illness and the necessity of being dependent upon others. In many ways it would resemble an HMO oriented to complete health care for the elderly, but it would differ from existing HMOs by being targeted only to older persons and by providing the types of services most often required by such persons—for example, home health care and nursing home care.

It must be recognized that this approach will require careful evaluation of many issues related to marketing, actuarial projections, identification of services to be included in the package, cost structure, and the extent of risk to be assumed by the policy holder.

4. Institutional Care Model

Nursing homes and hospitals are the acknowledged sites of institutional care. National guidelines for institutional care have been established by the Medicare and Medicaid programs. However, inasmuch as Medicaid is a state program, there are variations from state to state concerning the categories of licensed levels of care and reimbursement policies for each level of care.

Institutional care must deal with an important basic issue that differentiates it from the three types of living arrangement just described—namely, protection of personal privacy. Even in congregate housing, the resident can lock the door and maintain privacy within the apartment. This is not permissible in an institutional care setting.

Nursing Home Care. For the most part, there are three major categories of licensed nursing home care, with some states defining subcategories within these major units of *skilled, intermediate,* and *personal care.* Care may be provided on a short-term basis for posthospital and/or rehabilitation services, or it may be long-term chronic care of individuals not expected to return to their homes.

The nursing home is often capable of providing the most attentive, responsive, and intensive levels of chronic care and may for this reason be the preferred model for many individuals. Nursing homes can also offer specializations in services that are particularly intensive or difficult to provide at home.

Skilled care is defined by Medicare and Medicaid as that provided in a state-licensed institution (or a distinct part of an institution) that is primarily engaged in giving skilled nursing care and related services to patients who require medical, nursing, or rehabilitation services for an extended period of time but do not require hospitalization.

Intermediate care is that provided in an institution licensed by a state to provide health-related care to individuals who do not require the degree of care provided by a hospital or a skilled nursing facility but do require care or services available only through an institutional facility. These facilities are sometimes called supportive nursing care or health-related facilities.

Personal care is assistance with such activities of daily living as bathing, toileting, eating, transferring, and ambulating provided to an individual in an institutional setting. Customarily, three or more of these services are routinely provided to each client in order to qualify an institution as a personal-care facility. These institutions are also known as residential care facilities.

About 5 percent of the population aged 65 years and older lives in nursing homes. As was indicated earlier, in the population aged 85 and older, this is increased to 16 percent. Stated another way, 80 percent of persons living in nursing homes are individuals more than 85 years old.

Obviously, people are admitted to nursing homes because they cannot care for themselves or receive appropriate care at home. Some use nursing homes for posthospital rehabilitation and recuperation from the illness that required hospitalization.

Hospital Chronic Care. A prevailing myth in health care culture is that hospitals provide acute care and nursing homes provide chronic care. If this once was true, it certainly is the case no longer. Hospitals often treat people who have chronic illnesses. Hospital staff are sensitive to the needs of the chronically ill, even when the chronic illness is not the problem for which the patient is hospitalized.

Hospitals have great potential for innovative chronic care programs, because they are in a transition period during which their involvement in chronic care is increasing. As hospitals realize the appropriateness of their providing chronic care, the stage will be set for major changes in this arena.

Hospitals are evolving into institutions that deliver specific chronic care programs and may offer these either in the hospital or in other, nonhospital settings. This foray into the direct provision of new chronic care programs is what characterizes the change in hospital care. It is critical that hospitals not view acute and chronic care as mutually exclusive and recognize that chronic care can effectively be integrated into the fabric of the entire organization.

In Albuquerque, New Mexico, the Presbyterian Health Care system operates a nursing home adjacent to one of its hospitals. The nursing home offers skilled and intermediate care as well as care coordination to identify older hospital patients who could be enabled by coordinated chronic care services to remain at home rather than in a nursing home or hospital. The management of this nursing home, recognizing that these programs must be operated in their own style rather than replicating hospital procedures, has delegated responsibility for the chronic care system to administrators experienced in the delivery of chronic care services.

This has not precluded the nursing home from sharing many hospital services to its economic advantage. These include food services, housekeeping, maintenance, gardening, security, pharmacy, personnel, education, and central computing services. Such sharing, tailored to respond to the special needs of the nursing home, has eliminated the need to establish duplicate core functions and has provided economies of scale for the entire health care system.

The introduction of DRGs, with a resulting stimulus for earlier discharge of patients from acute care service, has combined with underutilization of hospital beds in many areas of the country and the growing numbers of older people to modify the role of the hospital.

Hospitals have converted unused beds to nursing home care and have developed a new level of care often called transitional care. These units are designed to provide transition from acute care to either nursing home care or home health care, and they often cater to patients requiring continued intensive rehabilitation, intensive surveillance, or the new high-technology feeding or respiratory services that are not available except in hospitals.

In some situations, especially in rural areas where there may be a short supply of institutional beds, the concept of "swing beds" has been introduced. A swing bed is one that can be used interchangeably as an acute care bed or a nursing home bed, depending on the care needs of the institution's current patient population. Unless a swing-bed provision has been established, however, it is not permissible to change the designation of the licensing of beds to meet changing patient demand.

As has been discussed earlier, some hospitals have developed a managed care program for older people that is designed to permit the hospital to provide or coordinate the delivery of care without the patient's having to be hospitalized.

As hospitals realize the appropriateness of their providing chronic care, the stage will be set for major changes in this arena, recognizing that:

1. Services should be modified to respond to the individual characteristics of the client.
2. Services should be respectful of the individual's cultural and religious beliefs and use that belief system to enhance the quality of care provided.
3. The client should have the right to reject any or all services.
4. The services should be arranged to normalize the client's life-style, accommodating timing and scheduling of delivery of services to the individual's preferences.

Organizational Formats for the Delivery of Chronic Care Services

While the chronic care system must be coordinated into a functional entity, the methods for achieving unity will vary with the community and its history and experiences in creating support for communitywide programs. A range of organizational format options exist, three of which are vertical integration, the brokered approach, and the federated approach.

The Vertical Integration Approach. A vertically integrated system can exist within the structure of an organized health care institution such as a hospital or may be designed as a free-standing system. Brody and Magel (1985) argue for the hospital's offering an array of services, because large numbers of persons are currently receiving ''step-down'' services, or services of diminished intensity, following hospitalization. These may include inpatient and outpatient rehabilitation services, convalescent care provided in nursing homes, home health care, and community outreach services. The hospital may already have many of the services represented in a vertically integrated system and be able to supplement them with new services to create a complete system. The hospital must, however, demonstrate that it has the philosophical and managerial orientation to respond appropriately in providing chronic care.

It would appear to be in the hospital's best interests to maintain the loyalty of an established clientele as well as the services it provides for its patients. In this integrated system, the patients will appreciate the convenience of a single organizational structure, the absence of the need to deal with multiple groups, and the simplicity of unified billing for all the services provided.

The Brokered Approach. In the brokered approach the coordinating agency usually retains some aspects of the core services (for example, assessment or care coordination) but contracts with other agencies to provide additional services. Some professionals prefer this model, because it encourages greater objectivity in assessment and care coordination; there is no pressure, overt or implied, to support services under the coordinating agency's auspices. The care coordinator can pick and choose from the services available throughout the community in order to design the most effective service package for the client.

While the services may be brokered from a variety of providers, the services to any user are coordinated by a single service—in other words, the agency provides care coordination. Here again, unified billing can be provided by the care coordination agency to simplify the process for the user.

The Federated Approach. Yet another approach to the management of a chronic care system is the federated approach, in which there is an alliance of chronic care services, whether freestanding or part of a larger organization. Within the federation the chronic care services become part of the organizational plan of the coordinating agency, sometimes referred to as a community care organization.

Each of the participants in this federation holds a position in a coordinating council that establishes common goals and methods of functioning. In this plan each participant retains the autonomy of its own organization but modifies its operational plan and policies to conform to the larger community organization. This plan obviously requires that each participating group forfeit some of its own visibility and identity for the greater good of the communitywide program. On the other hand, each participant gains from an enlarged source of referrals, participation in the growth of the communitywide organization, and avoidance of the need to develop duplicative services in order to establish a coordinated care system.

Existing services are used to their maximum capacity and additional overhead is avoided. However, individual agencies must submit to organizational plans imposed by others, and the advantages of a competitive market from which the coordinators may choose are reduced.

In this chapter some of the programs that are most frequently a part of a coordinated chronic care system have been described, along with some options for organizing these services into a coordinated system. It is unlikely that any program has been initiated with all of the services represented, yet many of the services do exist in a community and can be integrated into a program under the auspices of a potential sponsor of a coordinated chronic care system.

Chapter 5

THE ROLE
OF THE FAMILY

THOUGH THE TOPIC OF PARENT CARE excludes important aspects of family help to the old, it intimately concerns almost all of us who have had, now have or may in the future have a parent who is elderly, and all of us who have children and hope to grow old ourselves [Brody, 1985, p. 19].

Because most chronic care services are provided in the home, the primary environment of chronic care is the home and the family and community services available to persons living at home. Thus, a wide range of factors (including family, neighbors, and available community services) must be considered as significantly contributing to the care provided in the home environment. This does not negate the importance of the institution as a part of chronic care; it stresses only that institutional services should be viewed as augmenting the resources of the home and contributing an important component to the continuum of chronic care services.

While there are many and diverse influences on the environment of chronic care, the fact remains that the family is the primary source of care for the frail older person (Callahan,

71

Diamond, Giele, and Morris, 1980; Doty, 1986). Nearly three-fourths of the disabled older persons who do not live in institutions rely solely on family and friends, while most of the remainder depend upon a combination of family care and paid help (Soldo, 1983; Liu, Manton, and Liu, 1985).

Given the opportunity, most older persons suffering from some combination of chronic illnesses and functional impairment in the activities of daily living would prefer to continue to live at home, receiving care from "informal providers" (the term most often used to denote family members, neighbors, and friends who regularly provide care) and "formal providers" (the term used to denote professional or agency services provided for a fee).

Self-reliance and neighborly aid are traditional to the American way of life. This was particularly evident in our health care system during the early years of the United States, when neighbors and families nursed the sick and delivered babies.

Now, in the twentieth century, scientific progress has supplanted many of these home practices. Medical care has grown increasingly sophisticated, with professional caregiving being administered in well-equipped, sterile offices and hospitals.

However, highly specialized technical care is often criticized as being too impersonal and too costly. In fact, one of the most pressing social planning tasks of this and the coming decades revolves around the need to develop some type of coherent system of chronic care services for the elderly and the disabled. This system must include appropriate involvement of family members.

Caregiving is a universal experience and is not limited to one socio-economic, ethnic, or age group. All kinds of people are caregivers. The range and amount of care they provide also vary greatly.

The rewards of caregiving are primarily interpersonal. In addition to the enhancement of emotional ties, feelings of moral obligation and duty frequently underlie care. People's own early experiences, ethical standards, and religious values often determine how they will react to another's need for informal care.

The concept of *filial responsibility* refers to adults' obligations to meet their parents' basic needs. As a result of extensions in life expectancy, increasing numbers of parents and offspring are encountering the realities of this concept. Blenkner (1974) describes a "filial crisis" and the need of children to achieve "filial maturity." Difficulties may arise during a person's progress toward filial maturity, especially if inconsistencies exist between what parents and their offspring expect of one another or between what the individual perceives as approved by society and what that individual actually does.

Informal providers often labor under a lack of recognition and compensation. They are virtually ignored in Medicare, Medicaid, and disability insurance reimbursement mechanisms and in the planning and coordination of local service systems. In many arenas, strong economic and social disincentives work against the continuation of informal supports, to the detriment of the individuals involved and the cost to general taxpayers, who have to pay the bills for unnecessary or premature institutionalization.

The long-standing myth that portrayed the elderly as an isolated and abandoned population, without meaningful kin relationships, has been successfully destroyed in recent research. Far from abandoning the elderly, families, especially adult children, continue willingly to bear a major portion of caregiving. As Alvin Schorr (1980) writes, "The aged struggle against leaving home, and their families invest heavily in making it possible for them to stay" (p. 4).

A 1975 study found that four out of every five older persons had children. Of these, 18 percent lived in the household with a child and another 55 percent lived within thirty minutes of a child. Three-fourths (77 percent) had seen a child within the previous week (American Association of Retired Persons, 1985).

Repeatedly, studies have found that most older people are integral members of their family networks, that they see their adult children and other close kin at least several times a week, and that they interact regularly by telephone or letter with relatives who live far away.

When health and/or social assistance is needed, many elderly persons prefer to turn to their families and friends rather than to the formal service system. In general, families experience a pattern of reciprocal assistance between older and younger relatives, including economic and emotional aid, child care, household management, and health care. This pattern continues lifelong, but when elderly family members begin to need assistance, they start receiving more help than they give.

> Preliminary data from the Health Care Financing Administration's Long Term Care Survey demonstrates that, for the disabled population living in the community, relatives represent 84% of all caregivers for males and 79% for females. More wives than husbands care for disabled spouses, reflecting the fact that women outlive men by an average of seven years. More than one-third of all elderly disabled men living in the community are cared for by a wife, while only one in 10 disabled women is cared for by a husband.
>
> With increasing age, assistance given by spouses decreases as support from other family members and formal caregivers increases. Children of aging parents aged 85+ provide care to about one-third of elderly males and to slightly less than 40% of elderly females. Other relatives also are giving substantial care to elderly disabled family members aged 65+, representing 23% of all informal caregivers for men and 35% for women. For elderly females 85+, other relatives provide about 27% of all caregiving, while 36% of males in this group receive assistance from relatives other than a wife or children [U.S. Senate Special Committee on Aging, 1986, p. 96].

Recognition of the importance of family in the care of the chronically ill or disabled and the use of the home as the site where most chronic care services are delivered suggests that *families* should be viewed as the primary market for services that will enhance their capacity to provide care at home. Some concern has been expressed that when formal support services are available, especially those that are subsidized by public funds or covered by private chronic care insurance, they will be substituted for informal care by family and friends.

Results of a study of the National Channeling Demonstration Program (Stephens and Christianson, 1986) do not support this concern. Families' ability to maintain their informal care can be enhanced by the availability of appropriate education about the illness of the individual receiving care and ways the burden of giving adequate care can be reduced. Furthermore, programs that provide respite and/or peer support groups for caregivers increase the caregivers' capacity, skills, and willingness to perform the necessary tasks, even in the face of financial burdens or emotional stress. Also important is the awareness that additional resources will be available intermittently or continuously, if they are needed to enable the family to carry on its responsibilities as the primary caregiver.

To achieve the goals of family support, it becomes important for providers of services to become oriented to a family-centered configuration of chronic care and recognize that the family is the client, with each family member interacting with the chronic problems while participating in a response to the trajectory of needs of the afflicted person. In current practice, however, health care needs for service and eligibility for service are defined by the primary recipient of care.

It is this long-standing orientation to the provision of care that leads us to the view that family is outside the purview of the unit of care. At least, this is the perspective reinforced by the funding agencies, which do not usually acknowledge the significance of the family, the need to maintain family support, or the importance of providing care to family members.

What is needed is a paradigmatic shift to an orientation that considers the family as the unit of care and caring. This will require a fundamental change in the organization of insurance coverage, to make it possible for a family to purchase a policy under which it would receive benefits (including supportive services for the caregivers) that make it possible to care for a chronically ill older person.

Evidence that families already provide the major portion of chronic care in the manner most responsive to the needs of the frail individual is legion, and such care may be assumed by spouses, children, other relatives, or neighbors. However, it is usually a daughter who becomes the care provider (Brody, 1981). Because this situation has been clearly documented, it is obvious that to be most effective a chronic care system must respond to the needs of all caregivers, paying particular attention to ways these women can be helped to fulfill their often demanding role.

The magnitude of the share of chronic care of the frail elderly that is given by informal caregivers is dramatically shown in a national profile prepared from the 1982 National Long-Term Care Survey (Stone, Cafferata, and Sangl, 1987). The data from the survey revealed that:

- *The caregivers* were predominantly female (29 percent daughters and 23 percent wives), with 13 percent husbands. Their average age was 57.3, and one-quarter of them were aged 65 to 74; 10 percent were 75 or older. Approximately 70 percent were married; 54 percent of caretaking daughters were married, 14 percent were widowed, and 16 percent were divorced or separated. Over half of the caregivers (60 percent of the daughters and sons) lived with the care recipient. One-third of the caregivers worked outside the home. One-quarter of them reported having good health and one-quarter rated their health as fair or poor. One-third reported incomes at or near the poverty level. More than half of wives and husbands, 23 percent of daughters, and 11 percent of sons reported being sole providers of the household. One-third had no assistance in caring, 10 percent purchased services, and 29 percent were secondary caregivers.
- *Care recipients* had an average age of 77.7; 20 percent were 85 years old or older. Sixty percent were female. Half were married or widowed. Approximately 11 percent lived alone. One-third were poor or near poor, and 38 percent rated their health as poor. One-fifth reported no limitations on activities of daily living; 13 percent reported five or six such limitations. Twenty-nine percent reported three or fewer IADL

(instrumental activities of daily life) problems; 18 percent reported eight or nine such limitations. Caregiving was gender-linked: the major share was provided to females, and daughters and other female caregivers also were more likely than their male counterparts to be caring for an elderly woman.

- *Caregiver commitment* was intense. One-fifth of the caregivers had assumed the role for five years or longer, 44 percent had served from one to four years, and 18 percent had served for less than one year. Of the 16 percent who stopped providing care during the three-month interval between sample selection and interview, death of the recipient was the reason in one-half the instances, and one-fourth of the recipients had been institutionalized. Caregivers reported spending an average of four hours daily on caregiving tasks; for husbands, the average was five hours.

- *Caregiver tasks* also showed some gender-associated characteristics. Although two-thirds of caregivers helped with activities of daily living (feeding, bathing, dressing, and toileting), daughters were more likely to do so than sons. Of the 46 percent who helped the disabled person move about in the house or get out of bed, husbands were more likely to provide this service than were wives. Fifty-three percent of the caregivers administered medications; 86 percent spent extra time shopping for and/or transporting their relative. Extra time was spent performing household tasks by 80 percent of the caregivers. Men reported more time spent on chores such as meal preparation, housecleaning, and laundry. One-half the caregivers spent time handling family finances.

- *Competing demands* upon their time and energy were reported by one-fifth of all caregivers; one-quarter of the caregiving children had children under the age of 18 living at home. Nine percent had left the labor force to become a caregiver (13 percent of wives and 12 percent of daughters). Among the one million caregivers who had been employed at some time during the caregiver experience, 20 percent had cut back on hours, 29 percent had rearranged work schedules, and 19 percent had taken time off without pay.

- *Purchasers of services,* who made up less than 10 percent of the caregivers, were working primary caregivers, caregivers having high family income, or those caring for more severely impaired persons. Husbands were more likely than wives to purchase services.

In 1982 approximately 2.2 million caregivers aged 14 years or older were providing unpaid assistance to 1.2 million noninstitutionalized elderly disabled persons. With appropriate support, these helping persons can themselves be helped to avoid problems associated with the burdens of caregiving. If sufficiently strongly supported, they are able to continue to provide this help and to feel successful in the role of care provider.

The latter is important, because it is extremely damaging when family caregivers, faced with the changing needs of the primary client, feel that an unavoidable decline was in any way a product of failure or inadequacy on their part. This can be avoided by responding to the family members, or secondary clients, with respite from the continuous demands of caregiving, education to help them understand the course of the illness or disability and to enhance their skills, and interpersonal support through counseling. Just the knowledge that help is at hand if it should be needed is extremely helpful, even if that help is never called for.

One way that agencies can furnish support to secondary clients is through peer support groups. These may be organized informally by families seeking association with friends who have common problems or may be structured by health care providers as an ongoing resource to caregivers.

Some peer support groups take the form of mutual help groups, which have a widespread following. These are "characterized by small numbers of persons, mostly non-professionals, who want to meet on a regular basis for the purpose of sharing accounts of similar personal experiences, discussing coping strategies, engendering mutual support, and identifying and gaining access to community resources" (Haber, 1983, p. 251).

Other peer support groups are conducted by various national organizations. The Alzheimer's Disease and Related Disorders Association (ADRDA), for example, whose goals include family support, education, advocacy, and encouragement of research related to the understanding and cure of the disease, assists family members who are caring for individuals with Alzheimer's disease through local groups. These have been highly successful in a number of communities.

Yet another approach to the family support group is that which is agency supported, directed, and staffed. Clients are often referred to the group from other components of the care system because of a demonstrated high level of stress caused by overburdening responsibilities of caregiving. These groups may offer a formal curriculum and professional staff. An example of one such family support program is that sponsored by Pima County Aging and Medical Services and the Arizona Long Term Care Gerontology Center. It is illustrated by the following case study.

Case Study 12: A Neighborhood-Based Caregiver Network

Funding from the Administration on Aging and Pima County makes possible a project that brings together the resources of Pima County Aging and Medical Services and the Arizona Long Term Care Gerontology Center to complement the county's chronic care services with a special response to caregivers.

Groups are composed of from eight to ten participants and meet once a week for eight weeks, following a course outline that includes stress reduction, aging, nutrition, personal-care skills (for example, transferring, observing vital signs), behavior management, community helping resources, goal setting and action plans, and self-help. As the groups develop, members assume increasing responsibility for defining the workshop content.

During the eight-week period of project supervision, the emphasis of group meetings shifts from planning by staff toward planning by participants. It is expected that reinforcement of the caregivers' confidence in their expertise, growth of mutual support among members, and belief in the group's value will result from content that meets the members' needs.

The project is designed to assist each group to become self-sustaining after the eight-week period, no longer reliant on the support of project staff. This is accomplished through the increased involvement of participants in the planning of activities, through the affiliation of groups with local churches or community organizations, and through the provision of "booster workshops" to provide new incentives at three-month intervals after the eight-week initial period.

When these activities are accompanied by respite care for the patient, it is expected that family care will be sustained at a reduced stress level for the care providers.

Increasing awareness of the importance of family participation in the provision of chronic care should result in the development of family support activities that complement all the other chronic care services. As noted earlier, the *family* is the unit of care and must be acknowledged and supported in the delivery of chronic care.

Further reinforcement of the importance of family members' involvement in the provision of chronic care services will occur when public policies acknowledge the economic value of this support and provide some financial relief to families who care for their relatives in spite of economic hardship.

Doty (1986) lists a number of policy changes that have been suggested to promote family care at home: "These proposals include (1) tax incentives for family members who bring elderly impaired relatives into their homes, (2) public funding for 'respite' and other supportive services, (3) cash grants to low-income families to care for elderly relatives, (4) changes in supplemental security income (SSI) and food stamp rules such that benefits are not decreased when an elderly person moves in with a family, and (5) permitting family members to work as paid helpers under public programs" (p. 34). The expected effect of changed public policies "would be to reduce the negative consequences to families who have made a commitment to provide informal home care and would want to be able to continue this care" (p. 69).

Chapter 6

MODELS OF SUCCESSFUL
COORDINATED CARE PROGRAMS

MODELING IS THE PROCESS of creating a representation of any entity. Thus one might create a scale model of an airplane or a nursing home.

Modeling is a way of formulating relationships and exploring possible alternatives and outcomes. The value of a model to the social services researcher is not in its simplicity or complexity but rather in its appropriateness to the question of interest [Katzper, 1981, pp. 2-3].

Five programs that demonstrate the successful development of coordinated chronic care for the elderly have been selected as case illustrations for this book. They vary in their organizational structure, sponsorship, and funding, but all are effective. They are not the only programs of their type now operating in the United States, but their experiences show how existing resources can be consolidated to create an effective delivery system that responds to the needs of a particular community.

Each of these programs began with recognition by a local organization of deficiencies in medical and social services to the elderly. Each represents an innovative and imaginative integration of the efforts of established agencies and experienced professional personnel into a coordinated system that focuses on the individual as a whole person in a highly personal environment.

No one of the programs is likely to be duplicated exactly in another locale, but, having found workable solutions to some of the problems and challenges of chronic care, they are proof that the concept of a continuum of care is not just a theory. It is a practical approach that can be initiated by a health care agency, a hospital, or a government entity.

Case Study 13: On Lok Senior Health
Services (San Francisco, California)

On Lok is a nonprofit chronic care program that serves primarily Chinese, Italian, and Filipino residents within its neighboring area. Their average age is 80, and about two-thirds of them live alone. More than half do not speak English. All residents served by the program are certified for institutional long-term care by the California Department of Health Services as a condition of enrollment. In addition, On Lok cannot discharge participants and is responsible for their health care for the rest of their lives regardless of how sick they become.

Having started as one of the first day health programs in the country, the agency now operates three day health centers and On Lok House, a fifty-four-unit low-income housing facility for seniors. The comprehensive health program also includes in-home, hospital, and (when necessary) nursing home care for some 300 persons.

Joining the On Lok program is a three-part process: screening, assessment, and enrollment. First, the prospective participant and an On Lok social worker explore the program's features and eligibility requirements. Second, interested prospects who meet On Lok's frailty, age, and residency requirements receive a comprehensive health assessment by the program's multidisciplinary team. Third, a service plan is created.

On Lok's multidisciplinary team includes physicians, nurses, social workers, nutritionists, therapists, paraprofessionals, and other support staff. Unlike the more common brokerage programs, not only does On Lok's team assess participants and develop individual treatment plans, but its staff directly delivers and formally reassesses clients quarterly. This consolidated approach for the very impaired results in a more responsible system with lower case management costs. Together, this team provides primary medical care; dental care; skilled nursing care; physical, occupational, and recreational therapies; social services; nutritional counseling; medical day care; social day care; postdischarge planning; pharmacy services; all health-related transportation; and some in-home services. Essentially, in return for its monthly capitation premium, On Lok pays for and provides every health and health-related service from transportation and social support to acute hospitalization. And most of these services are provided directly by On Lok staff. Care by professional medical specialists, institutional care (acute and skilled nursing), and medical specialty services are provided under contract.San Francisco: Jossey-Basstudy 14

On Lok is the only long-term care program in the country receiving capitation financing from Medicare, Medicaid, and private individuals, and assuming full financial risk. On Lok's unique service program is made possible through Medicare 222 and Medicaid 1115 waivers. The waivers are normally time limited; but in spring 1986, federal legislation was passed to make these waivers for On Lok permanent. Perhaps the most interesting development is the national replication of On Lok's financing model. Many people have expressed interest in (but question) the generalizability of the model. In the fall of 1986, federal legislation was passed to extend this financing model and its waivers to ten other sites around the country.

Case Study 14: St. Vincent's Hospital and Medical Center of New York

The Department of Community Medicine at St. Vincent's conducts two distinct long-term home health care programs for the frail aged in the hospital's community. The Chelsea-Village Program (CVP), so designated because St. Vincent's serves the areas of Greenwich Village and Chelsea in Manhattan, has been in operation since 1973, bringing physician–nurse–social worker teams to the homes of older homebound persons. In the past fifteen years about 16,000 home visits have been made to about 1,500 individuals whose average age is 83. Two-thirds are women. Two-thirds live alone. All are bound to home by chronic illness and frailty. The active caseload of the CVP is about 160 persons. Eligibility requirements are simple: patients must be homebound, be reasonably reachable geographically, lack effective access to other service providers at home, and be willing to receive the St. Vincent's team. There exists no financial eligibility requirement, and all services are given free to patients. No reimbursement is obtained from patients or families, nor does Medicare or Medicaid pay. The CVP is supported by the hospital and by private philanthropy.

The New York State Medicaid-funded nursing home without walls program was initiated in 1979, and the Department of Community Medicine at St. Vincent's was one of the first pilots. This program is distinguished from the CVP by its broad array of in-home services, including not only the physician–nurse–social worker team but also various therapies, paraprofessional care, medical equipment and supplies, nutritional counseling, heavy chore services, and personal emergency response systems. Only persons entitled to Medicaid are eligible, with few exceptions, and the patient's rights to remain eligible are held to rigid norms of cost and service. The St. Vincent's Program has an active case roster of about eighty patients.

The fact that both programs are available to the elderly in the hospital's general area creates what is in effect a comprehensive system of long-term home health care for the aged, under the auspices of a single organization. St. Vincent's can draw upon a wide variety of services to meet specific needs of any patient at any time, regardless of the individual's financial status.

Case Study 15: Mount Zion Hospital and
Medical Center (San Francisco, California)

The San Francisco Institute on Aging is a community-based, comprehensive health care center dedicated to fostering health and well-being among elderly citizens of San Francisco. The institute is a subsidiary of Mount Zion Health Systems, Inc., along with Mount Zion Hospital and Medical Center. Mount Zion has been a leader in geriatric care for the past thirty years.

Mount Zion Hospital and Medical Center, a nonprofit community hospital, has 439 acute care beds, 31 skilled nursing facility beds, and 8 geriatric assessment and rehabilitation beds. The San Francisco Institute on Aging and Mount Zion Hospital serve 5,000 patients each year, which translates into about 50,000 patient contacts annually.

The institute has more than seventeen different programs and together with the hospital serves 15 to 20 percent of the elderly market share in San Francisco (a total population of 735,000, with about 16.5 percent elderly).

The San Francisco Institute on Aging serves as an umbrella organization that incorporates the spectrum of services that constitute a continuum of care. Included in the continuum are traditional inpatient, outpatient, and skilled nursing services. The service system is designed to maintain maximum functional independence for seniors with a wide range of needs. Client transition between services is facilitated by the presence of all types of services either within a single organization or available to the organization through contracts with other community service agencies. Coordination and integration of services within the continuum occur through assessment, care coordination, and interdisciplinary teamwork. Coordination between the formal services and informal services provided by family and friends is critical.

The focal program for the hospital-based long-term care initiative is the Mount Zion Care Account, an organizational entity that manages the delivery of a comprehensive package of geriatric services to elderly participants by coordinating inpatient, outpatient, and geriatric services. The service coordinator or nurse advocate is the pivotal component within the arranged care system.

The program is designed for 2,000 Medicare beneficiaries who have Medicare supplemental insurance and are willing to use Mount Zion Hospital and Mount Zion Medical Group participating physicians.

There is no charge for becoming a member of Mount Zion Care Account, and this preferred provider organization (PPO) provides for more services at less out-of-pocket expense than does the traditional system. Participating providers, including 160 private physicians representing all specialties, have contracted with the Mount Zion Care Account to accept assignments and process Medicare and insurance claims. This service results in reduced paperwork and increased reimbursement coverage for the participants.

Other services, available at reduced rates, include:

- Adult day health care
- Home health care (rehabilitation and maintenance)
- Geriatric assessment service
- Geriatric inpatient rehabilitation and assessment
- Artworks
- Lifeline (emergency response system)
- Senior companion program
- Alzheimer's day care
- Dental care
- Prescriptions
- Eye and vision care
- Hearing and audiology services
- Transportation
- Health screening
- Health insurance counseling
- Skilled nursing facility

Future plans include the use of a chronic care data base to establish the efficiency of a chronic care insurance product or prepaid wraparound. Since the health environment is changing so rapidly in San Francisco, including the presence of many empty acute care hospital beds, it is difficult to predict need far into the future. Mount Zion Hospital is in the process of downsizing, yet it is expanding its geriatric service component through the San Francisco Institute on Aging.

Case Study 16: Sinai Samaritan
Medical Center (Milwaukee, Wisconsin)

Hospital-based care coordination is a recent development and constitutes a new role for institutions fostering continuity of care. This new role encompasses the coordination and monitoring of health and social services, including in-home service providers, to reduce fragmented care. Continuity of care in this new institutional role is further enhanced by provision of ongoing, specialized medical care in addition to care coordination.

In 1983 Sinai Samaritan Medical Center established the Geriatrics Institute, Mount Sinai campus, which focuses on patient care, research, and education and emphasizes helping older adults maintain their independence. Its multidisciplinary staff of geriatricians, geriatrics-trained nurse specialists, rehabilitation therapists, and social service professionals provides comprehensive health and social services for older adults and their families. The range of inpatient and outpatient services includes an outpatient clinic and four community-based wellness clinics, an acute care unit, outpatient and inpatient geropsychiatry, Alzheimer's disease and rehabilitation day care programs, family support and education programs, a geriatric team consultation service (inpatient and physicians' outreach), and a care coordination system.

The Geriatrics Institute was awarded a grant during its first year of operation from the Robert Wood Johnson (RWJ) Foundation Program for Hospital Initiatives in Long-Term Care. This grant enabled the Geriatrics Institute to develop a continuum of care that provides innovative patient services, a comprehensive data system, and an efficient care coordination system.

The care coordination system provides hospital-based case management services to the frail elderly enrolled in outpatient and inpatient programs. Frail elderly adults (the average patient age is 76) in need of care coordination/case management services typically have multiple chronic diseases with resulting disabilities that require in-home support services to allow the elderly continued independent living. Care coordination/case management systems are designed to assess the client's needs, to develop and implement a care plan, and to coordinate and monitor the necessary institutional and community-based services that help support the older adult's independence.

The institute's care coordination model incorporates the institute's own direct services and brokers community resources to provide comprehensive care for its clients. In this model the care coordinator coordinates, monitors, and advocates on behalf of the client needing ambulatory services, in-home formal services, and informal family supportive care. Care coordination is available to frail, acute care, and ambulatory patients with functional impairments and poor social resources. A computerized data system assists in the development of service plans and facilitates the monitoring of ongoing care.

The care coordination system has four phases: case finding, care plan development, initiation of services, and follow-up monitoring and evaluation. The results of a comprehensive assessment inventory completed by a registered nurse, social worker, and physician provide the data base for eligibility. The case finding (or screening) for eligible clients occurs during the daily interdisciplinary staff conference held for all new acute care or ambulatory patients. Since care coordination is targeted toward the frail or older adult at risk of institutionalization, criteria have been established to identify eligible individuals. After eligibility has been determined, a case manager is assigned to coordinate institute- and community-based resources.

The care coordinator and the multidisciplinary team identify the problems to be addressed and develop a preliminary care plan. Finalization of the plan is completed by the care coordinator, who initiates services in conjunction with the discharge department of the medical center. Follow-up and monitoring occur on a biweekly or monthly basis, with reevaluation occurring every six months. This monitoring and evaluation process includes identifying patient progress, the level of service utilization, and the appropriateness of the care plan. Dialogue with community service providers assures that care-coordinated patients receive appropriate in-home services.

The model is administered by the care coordination supervisor, who is responsible for system development and assures care plan implementation. The care coordinators are nurses and social workers who provide direct care in the diverse components of the institute. These multidisciplinary care coordinators maintain small caseloads of clients in addition to their ongoing work responsibilities.

Integration of a care coordination system into an acute care institution requires changes in the internal and external roles and services traditionally associated with hospitals. At the Geriatrics Institute, the implementation process was carefully planned to involve hospital personnel. A committee composed of representatives of the pertinent hospital departments and institute staff was organized to address the concerns of key personnel in the evolution of the model. The role of the care coordinator was extensively discussed, thus minimizing "turf issues" with other professionals involved in discharge planning. Identification of how and when the care coordination system would become involved in patient management also helped neutralize the territorial issues associated with new hospital programs. Inservice programs were implemented for social work and nursing staff on both the inpatient and outpatient units. A pilot program was conducted for one month to allow the care coordination staff the opportunity to put into operation, evaluate, and modify the model prior to formal implementation. The pilot program also allowed the hospital staff an opportunity to influence the final model. (For more information see Olson, Prochnow, and Zalenko, 1986.)

Case Study 17: Pima County Aging
and Medical Services (Tucson, Arizona)

Pima County Aging and Medical Services provides both institutional and home-based care. Skilled nursing home care is offered to persons meeting established financial eligibility standards at the county-owned Posada del Sol Nursing Home and other licensed facilities throughout the community.

The county does its own assessment of persons entering its system. All in-home services are provided through contracts with community agencies that hold the appropriate license to do so. These include:

Service	*Provider*
Assessment	Pima County
Case management	3 private family service agencies
Home care	Private home care agencies
Adult day care	Handmaker Geriatric Center
Home-delivered meals	Title III (OAA) Meals
Socialization/nutrition	Title III (OAA)
Chore service	Title III (OAA) and Title XX (SSBG)
Lifeline (emergency response system)	Title III (OAA)
Shopper service	Title XX (SSBG)

To pay for its coordinated care system, Pima County combines funds received from a number of funding sources. Community-based services are funded primarily by Social Services Block Grants, Title III, state supplemental payments, the city of Tucson, United Way, Pima County, foundation contributions, and private donations. Alternative residential services draw resources from Pima County, private donations and client contributions, HUD Section 8, and Title 19 (medical care only). Nursing home care (both contracted and in the county-owned Posada del Sol) is supported by Pima County, client contributions, state supplemental payments, third-party payers, and Title 19 (medical care only).

All five of these programs began with a realistic analysis of health care limitations in their home communities. Each then moved on to define a specific goal that it was qualified to seek and put together an imaginative program that makes the most of whatever resources are available to it.

Chapter 7

PLANNING A
COORDINATED CARE SYSTEM

MANY OF US MAY SIMPLY NEED to reorient the way we think about care of the elderly—society needs to re-examine how it pays for care. Caring is hard work; it is no less demanding than learning to remove a cataract, no less taxing to the individual practitioner than the operating table, no less valuable than managing or insinuating a catheter, and no less significant to patients' lives than technically sophisticated appliances. We need to recognize the importance of alternative modes of caring which include a range of strategies, both medical and non-medical, delivered within and outside of hospitals [Eisdorfer, 1985, p. 579].

While chronic care services can be offered in a variety of settings, under a variety of sponsorships, and for different populations, it is helpful to structure a framework for planning that is consistent with generic planning approaches yet specific to chronic care. The framework makes it possible to view all of the options and variables in order to identify how to begin the program and shape its growth. Such a plan is the best way to ensure that the major services are included and to provide the flexibility to accommodate to individual differences among clients. The special characteristics of each program and its relationship to the community are similarly protected by a carefully structured framework. A chronic care program that is to be comprehensive will, after providing the initial assessment and care coordination, provide options for services in a variety of settings.

Major steps to be undertaken in the establishment of a coordinated chronic care system are displayed in the following list:

1. *Establish Future Direction*
   Articulate philosophy
   Formulate mission statement

2. *Plan Strategies*
   Assess internal strengths/weaknesses
   Identify obstacles
   Determine financial resources
   Evaluate community resources

3. *Evaluate Existing Market*
   Target market segments
   Assess competitive position

4. *Assess Alternatives*
   Do nothing/reassess the mission statement
   Co-opt other services
   Enter into a joint venture
   Establish a vertically integrated system

Establish Future Direction

Establishment of future direction begins with statements of philosophy and mission that articulate the direction that will be taken in the next steps in the planning process.

Articulate Philosophy. A statement of philosophy should express the values of the sponsoring organization. This statement should guide the development of a long-range plan and the implementation of services in order to provide the organization with a sense of cohesion and coherence to guide its efforts and a framework within which to assess the evolution of the program in response to changing needs and service capacities. The philosophy might read something like this:

> Recognizing that older people are as diverse as society as a whole, we are committed to respect for the individual. Our programs will serve older persons who are well, as well as those who are ill. We will attempt to enhance each individual's sense of well-being and help him or her retain the highest degree of independence possible.
>
> We consider chronic care to be more than medical care for the chronically ill older person. In addition, we will include a wide range of social and psychological supportive services for the individual and the family unit to which he or she belongs.
>
> Whenever possible, we will attempt to help a frail or disabled person remain at home by providing services there. When the home no longer can offer the necessary therapeutic environment, we will recommend institutional care only after a complete assessment of the person's needs has been completed. We will involve the individual and family members to the greatest degree possible in any decision to seek institutional care.
>
> As part of our role in our home community, we will participate in outreach programs designed to identify persons in need of services and will cooperate to the fullest extent possible with other service providers.

Formulate Mission Statement. Clarification and enunciation of the values and philosophy of a coordinated chronic care system make it possible to formulate a succinct mission statement such as the following: "This comprehensive service program is designed to address the needs of a wide variety of older persons throughout the community and will incorporate agencies that already exist, coordinating their delivery and supplementing them with additional services that are required to create a continuum of care."

Plan Strategies

The organization that is considering becoming the developer of a chronic care program should learn all it can about the kinds of services that should be included as appropriate to chronic care. It can achieve this goal by reviewing the literature related to the identified area of chronic care, subscribing to the relevant journals, attending conferences and workshops, and making on-site visits to or tours of existing programs that have established reputations for leadership and quality of services. The discussion in Chapter Six of five exemplary chronic care programs may provide the initial introduction to a program of particular interest.

While it is costly for a large group of planners or policy makers to travel some distance to view a program, an alternative approach might be to invite someone from each of several programs considered promising models to come to the proposed location of a new program to offer an intensive workshop for a large group of the people who will be involved.

It will also be important to determine what the competition is doing and what has been successful in comparable situations. It is not, however, feasible to develop a program predicated solely upon the activities of others. It will be more valuable to look within and to build upon the strengths discovered in one's own organization, coordinating those strengths to make them relevant and supplementary to all the services currently provided in the community.

Assess Internal Strengths/Weaknesses. It will therefore be useful to conduct an inventory of internal strengths, resources, and possible weaknesses as well as other resources available in the community. This may be accomplished by engaging external consultants or by making a conscientious self-study. In either case, the major considerations should include:

- An inventory of services currently provided by the potential sponsor that are oriented toward meeting the needs of the older population.

- A listing of the advantages to the sponsor of providing these services.
- A realistic determination of whether these specialty services are essential components of the organization.
- An analysis of whether or not existing specialty services can be integrated into a comprehensive program. Are there any obstacles to the expansion or integration of these services? List all the advantages of expanding these services.
- A listing of key personnel within the sponsoring organization who have special expertise in services to the elderly.
- A determination of the visions of persons so identified for the development of a coordinated care system. Are these persons available to provide leadership to this program?
- An analysis of conflicting priorities that might distract from services to the elderly.

Candid analysis of the data drawn from this examination will generate a profile of the status of chronic care in the possible sponsor's organization and suggest what approaches offer the most promise of increasing the scope of chronic care services.

The following hypothetical illustrations show what such a profile might look like and what it might reveal.

Case Study 18: Profile Sample 1

Glenborough Hospital has 200 beds and is located in a small metropolitan area. Although it may be described as a community hospital, providing a range of medical-surgical services, it has developed a special reputation for its rehabilitation services. It has an aggressive physical therapy department, recently expanded, and has engaged an occupational therapist and a speech pathologist on a contractual basis. In turn, the rehabilitation program has contracted to provide rehabilitation services to three nursing homes. The hospital participates in a hospital-based home health care agency and conducts an annual health screening program for the local senior center.

- *Current services.* Inpatient hospital care, rehabilitation services, and health screening.
- *Strengths.* The rehabilitation services have stimulated high utilization by older persons, with resultant high occupancy and profitability for the hospital.
- *Weaknesses.* The hospital provides no follow-up coordination of its rehabilitation services with services its patients receive at home or in clinics after discharge. There is no coordination with the home health service.
- *Reasons for expansion.* Rehabilitation services are important to the older person, are in short supply, and are a critical part of qualifying for reimbursement for nursing home and home care. Glenborough can develop a unique role locally in providing services for the elderly.

  Beginning associations have been established with home health care services and with the local senior center. What is needed now is a coordinated system that integrates the services into a comprehensive program.

  One of the social workers, who minored in gerontology in graduate school and has shown a special affinity for developing programs for older people, is concerned about the absence of coordination of services after the patient leaves the hospital.

  A local community foundation has expressed interest in supporting hospital initiatives in chronic care and has invited proposals to generate a demonstration program.
- *Summary.* The hospital's rehabilitation focus, the presence of an understanding staff, and experiences in the community all suggest it would be desirable for the hospital to develop an integrated chronic care service system that will build upon the rehabilitation services, provide coordinated care, and contract for some services with other community organizations.

Case Study 19: Profile Sample 2

Riverview Manors is a small group of nursing homes concentrated in one sector of a populous northern state. The homes are located in both rural and metropolitan areas, take advantage of group purchasing and centralized accounting, and have nursing care consultation from administrative headquarters. Riverview Manors' facilities provide two levels of nursing home care and include one adult day health care program. The firm, which enjoys a good reputation for quality institutional care, is looking ahead and trying to forecast its future in the community. It appears possible that its role as a leader in chronic care is being eroded by the hospitals and home health care agencies. While Riverview's status seems secure for the present, its administrators are sensitive to changing trends in health care nationwide; they fear that unless they maintain an aggressive and innovative position, they will lose their market share and leadership in the communities where they operate.

- *Current services.* Skilled and intermediate levels of nursing home care and adult day health care services.
- *Strengths.* The group's staff members possess great skill and knowledge in the provision of chronic care and are capable of supporting additional chronic care activities.

  Development of a coordinated chronic care system would permit expansion into home-delivered services and additional day health care centers. These would increase the income base and broaden the potential market. What is now a small group of nursing homes could in this way become the primary community care coordination agency for persons able to pay for the services they require.
- *Weaknesses.* There is limited follow-up of patients after discharge from the nursing homes and too much dependence on hospitals for referrals to the nursing homes and the day health care program.
- *Summary.* The great strengths of this group lie in its community reputation, skilled staff, and competence to provide a variety of chronic care services. Stability and comfort in the past have led this successful nursing home group into a complacency that recently has been challenged by the increased competitiveness of chronic care services and widespread recognition of a growing market. Riverview Manors is ready to develop a coordinated chronic care system.

Identify Obstacles. While many strengths that will support entry into a chronic care program should be evident in the organization, it would be foolhardy to overlook obstacles to a successful program.

For example, there may be competing interests within the organization that will preclude the chronic care program's receiving the support essential to assure its success. It may be perceived that chronic care is the domain of other groups and that venturing into the arena would present unnecessary competition with services already being provided.

The ability to develop new programs may depend upon the availability of competent staff, so a shortage of needed personnel could be a real obstacle to a new venture.

In some situations the regulatory requirements of a certificate of need, license, or zoning approval may prove formidable impediments to the development of some portions of the program.

Determine Financial Resources. Not the least of apparent obstacles will be the need to ensure that there is adequate financing to initiate the new venture and maintain a high level of service.

Evaluate Community Resources. If the organization has not heretofore been in the chronic care business, it may have access to some of the critical resources and at the same time lack adequate capacity to transfer those resources easily to a chronic care program. Of itself, this limitation should not be a major deterrent, if the organization is in a position to coordinate its resources with the strengths of other community organizations to achieve such capacity through collaboration with others. In order to determine what community resources already exist and how they might augment those of the primary organization, communitywide resource evaluation should be conducted as the next step. The information sought should include:

- A listing of all services for the older population that could be provided through contracts with other organizations. Can these services be expanded? Can they be integrated into a coordinated system of chronic care?
- A listing of the advantages to the sponsoring organization

of contracting for such services. A similar listing of disadvantages.

- A listing of organizational contacts the sponsoring organization already has with other agencies serving the elderly, especially the state and area agencies on aging, and membership or advocacy groups.
- A listing of other persons elsewhere in the community who might be available to provide leadership for the program.
- Determination of whether a university-based center on aging is available to provide support services for the project.

Case Study 20: Brookhurst Hospital

Brookhurst Hospital wished to intensify its services to the elderly but felt it had insufficient expertise to jump into new program development. In a move to correct this situation, the hospital administration asked its vice-president for planning to attend meetings of the local Council on Aging.

At one of these meetings it was pointed out that the community had no adult day health program, and a discussion of the possible development of such a program ensued. During this dialogue the Brookhurst vice-president offered an unused area of the hospital as a program site, and the offer was immediately accepted by the council.

As a result, an adult day health center quickly evolved and the hospital entered into a contract to provide meals and some limited staff services to the new program. The vice-president for planning became a regular participant in the council's activities.

In the following year the council planned a health fair and invited the hospital to be host and cosponsor of this community program. The hospital thus, in a relatively short time, established itself as an important participant in the provision of aging services in the community.

Evaluate Existing Market

Having established the goals and purposes of the organization, and having assessed its strengths and weaknesses and assured the availability of funds, the next step is to evaluate the existing market, the services currently available, and opportunities for the organization. It is important at this point to recall and appreciate the heterogeneity of the aging market. For example, if the term *the elderly* is defined as encompassing all persons aged 65 and older, it may apply to an age distribution far too wide to permit valid generalization. Exploration of the market should therefore take into consideration more specific age groups and target them by such characteristics as place of residence, income, degree of chronic conditions experienced, limitations of activities of daily living, availability of social supports, access to services, and religious or social group affiliations. Obviously, an important factor in market assessment is the ability to determine as accurately as possible the concerns and interests of the particular group the organization hopes to serve.

Target Market Segments. An illustration of the importance of appropriate targeting of a potential market can be found in the evolution of congregate housing for the elderly. At one time considered to be primarily a service for persons requiring financial assistance, it now also serves those who have substantial incomes sufficient to meet sizable entrance fees and monthly service charges. Between these two extremes lies a large segment of the population with varying financial capacities and interest in committing a large share of resources to this kind of service.

In an estimate of the size of the potential elderly market, it is not sufficient simply to enumerate numbers of persons by age category. Financial capacity and interest in a particular lifestyle must also be explored. Will the program proposed be targeted to the younger or the older portion of the general category of "elderly"? It should be remembered that the older the population served, the more important it will be to make health services available. Conversely, if such health services are promoted, the more attractive the program will be to persons who are very old and may require increasing health care with the onset of chronic problems.

In addition to financial issues and age and health status, other concerns will include current living arrangements, the geography of the community or subsection thereof, and the proximity of the proposed service to a supportive social network of family or other close associates. A potential client's decision to select a particular service may be influenced by the availability of public or special needs transportation or by the capacity of the individual to own and drive a car.

Some persons will be attracted to a program with a specific religious orientation, creating a special market niche related to sponsorship by a religious group.

An additional feature, especially important in the development of an institutional program, is the location. For example, it is unlikely that a downtown location adjacent to a hospital would attract early retirees to a congregate housing development. They would find a site beside a golf course, lake, or beach much more attractive. The level of service can be dictated by the site's location.

Not the least of the issues related to defining various market segments and selecting which to target is potential clients' perceptions of their own needs, capacities, and limitations, and their perceptions of how the availability of a given service may enhance their ability to remain self-sufficient. Will the service be one that gives clients a greater sense of independence and self-worth?

The inventory of community services should incorporate an exploration of their capacity to serve as part of a coordinated system and of their compatibility with the potential sponsoring organization's goals. In addition, it should identify service gaps and agencies that may be expected to remain competitors.

Each of the relevant concerns should be examined in the context of a specific market segment, rather than the thirty-year range that constitutes the entire elderly segment of the population. For example, it will not be sufficient to count the number of adult day health care programs available in a community in order to determine whether additional services of this type may be required. The existing services may be specifically oriented toward the developmentally disabled person receiving public support and having transportation available. Such a program would probably not contribute to a comprehensive care system serving the aging, nor would an existing day health care program serving only persons able to pay the full cost of services.

A valuable tool in the exploration of appropriate market segments to be served is the use of *focus groups,* small discussion groups that provide input on a given project during its planning stages. The composition of the focus groups should closely approximate that of the market segment being explored. For example, if the intention is to discover the response of early retirees to a new insurance program, it would not be helpful to include chronically ill persons in their eighties and nineties.

Consider the following example: A Catholic diocese planned to build a new congregate housing program on a parcel of land it had obtained in a newly developing area of the town. A new parish church was also proposed on the same plat, once the population was estimated to be sufficiently large. A group of Catholics from the downtown area served by the diocesan cathedral were invited to discuss design, program, and fees. These participants refused to discuss the issues placed on the agenda, because they rejected the site as being too far from their neighborhood. They wanted housing within walking distance of the cathedral.

Obviously this was the wrong focus group to select for obtaining input on this project. Participants should have been from the area of the proposed housing—but that was unfortunately not possible, because residents of this area did not include elderly persons.

Assess Competitive Position. A comprehensive analysis of the market should also analyze the competitiveness of the new product with existing and proposed programs and should provide recommendations for future action. A market evaluation should include:

- Identification of any strong competitors already providing a chronic care program.
- Identification of special demonstration programs or grant-supported programs in chronic care that are currently functioning in the community. Has the sponsoring organization any relationship with such programs?

- Identification of any planned or proposed projects that might compete in the same market, the scope of their proposed service packages, and the timetables for their development. This is one of the most difficult undertakings to describe accurately, because in unregulated services such as housing there is no formal requirement for identification of planned programs.

A typical table of contents for a market survey report, shown in Table 5, suggests what the exploration should encompass.

Table 5. Market Survey Report Table of Contents.

Introduction	i
Definition of Services	1
General Population Trends	8
Service Area Analysis	17
Population Trends	17
Income Characteristics	23
Inventory of Services	33
Focus-Group Discussions	37
Program Plan and Recommendations	41
Timeline	45

An outgrowth of such a study should include the identification of alternative market opportunities, with an evaluation of the positive and negative aspects of each option.

Assess Alternatives

At this point, before the organization is ready to proceed with implementation of strategies, several alternatives should be considered: do nothing/reassess the mission, co-opt other services, enter into a joint venture, or establish a vertically integrated system.

As part of the assessment of alternatives, the sponsor is encouraged to evaluate groups targeted for service and to delineate the proposed services carefully. For example, as noted earlier, it is not adequate to target services to the elderly without also defining the age, health status, income, and dependency of clients to be served. The more precise the target group, the easier it will be to design an appropriate program and to market it successfully.

Selecting an area of service and a target market permits continued exploration of the resources essential for the effective implementation of the program. First of all, it will be essential to have adequate personnel who possess the requisite skills. A community study may have indicated that a rehabilitation program is the highest-priority chronic care need in a particular area, while a personnel survey may have shown not only that there are no physiatrists in the community but that an intensive two-year search for other rehabilitation specialists was unsuccessful. The reason for the lack of a rehabilitation program is then clear, but before it is possible to proceed with plans for one, it will be necessary to mount a plan for recruiting the necessary personnel. Until this problem can be resolved, inauguration of this type of service has to be postponed.

Any venture will also require a considerable amount of start-up capital and other financial support. The sponsor must ask which alternative represents a project to which it wishes to dedicate the finite funds it has available.

Do Nothing/Reassess the Mission Statement. One alternative is to do nothing additional in chronic care—to maintain the status quo. To assume this posture will not be difficult if the initial assessment clearly indicates the wisdom of such a decision. There might, however, be a plan to update the study at a later date to see if changes warrant subsequent reconsideration.

Some questions that arise may be helpful in determining whether or not to proceed. Among these may be uncertainty about whether or not the proposed program is compatible with the mission of the sponsoring group. The evolution of recommendations based on the market analysis may point to a need not considered when the study was initiated. It is important to ask whether the program and the population are harmonious with the goals of the sponsor. If not, the sponsor must decide whether it is prepared to restate its mission to make it consistent with needs made evident by the study, a dilemma illustrated by the following case study.

Case Study 21: Downtown Hospital

Downtown Hospital commissioned a study to select a site and prepare for the development of a nonsubsidized housing program. The hospital claimed that it had had poor experiences with government-sponsored programs and wished to move into the private-pay market.

A study conducted by a consultant for the hospital pointed out the enormous capital investment that would be required, the anticipated impact upon the hospital's borrowing capacity, the substantial vacancy rates of numerous privately owned congregate housing developments, and the existence of long waiting lists for subsidized housing in the community.

After examining several options, the hospital trustees acknowledged that the mission of the religiously oriented hospital made it more appropriate for them to apply for federal funds for a subsidized housing program. The application was successful and the housing was built.

The hospital could have changed its mission had its trustees so desired, but having access to a mission statement as well as to the alternative development possibilities helped them to choose the course they believed best for them at the time. Choosing the alternative it did in no way precluded Downtown Hospital's developing nonsubsidized housing at another time.

Co-Opt Other Services. If a decision is made to proceed, there are at least three possible alternatives. One is development of a comprehensive program by co-opting or taking over existing services, without adding new services. For example, an HMO might assume ownership of several disparate parts of a community chronic care program and combine them with the physician, rehabilitation, assessment, and home health services it already offers. A hospital might purchase a home health care agency and nursing home, thereby putting together the critical parts of a chronic care system that would require only the addition of assessment and care coordination to become complete.

Enter into a Joint Venture. Another approach could be a joint venture, in which the sponsor shares development risks and opportunities with another community group (or groups). For example, a hospital might enter into a joint venture with a nursing home and a home health care agency to develop the rudiments of a coordinated comprehensive chronic care program (see Figure 8).

Figure 8. ABC Chronic Care Program.

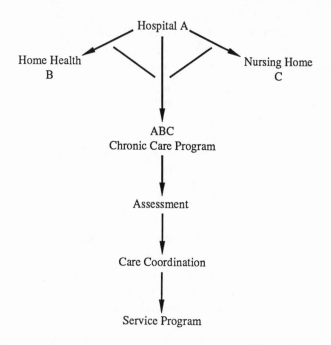

Case Study 22: Southside Hospital

Southside Hospital, located in an area having a dense population of older people, had given careful consideration to enlarging its services to the community and concluded that the development of a care coordination program would serve both its own needs and those of the community in the best possible way.

The hospital fully intended that its new program be clearly identified as a service to the community, but when plans for implementation were developed it was learned that the local Area

Agency on Aging had plans to offer a similar care coordination system. This created the dilemma of having to decide whether to proceed independently, to compete with the area agency and thereby possibly create an antagonistic environment, or to find some way of avoiding conflict.

After a series of meetings between the hospital and the agency to explore the possibility of their working together, it was recognized that the hospital had financial resources and the area agency had close contacts and a trusting relationship with many older persons. Each group reassessed its goals and mission and decided neither would be compromised by entering into a joint venture, which was then arranged.

Joint ventures are effective when each participant brings an important aspect of the program to the relationship, has a clear understanding of the expectations of the relationship, and is capable of realizing its share of these expectations.

In some situations the joint venture may be an interim arrangement, lasting only until a new and stable organizational plan that will be less cumbersome and more responsive to program needs can be evolved.

Case Study 23: The Teaching Hospital

A major health care foundation offered to fund the planning for an innovative approach to the delivery of chronic care services, but the requirements for proposals seeking such support were so complicated that an interested teaching hospital invited three other groups to participate in a joint venture for the purpose of devising a program that would be competitive. All four components of the joint venture entered into it understanding that their affiliation in the project was a temporary expedient and that a less cumbersome and more efficient management plan for implementation of the program would evolve as their efforts progressed.

The situation just described illustrates how joint ventures may be used to meet new organizational goals without commitment to this joint structure over an extended period. In some situations the joint venture may be the forerunner of a planned, intended takeover by a single organization.

Case Study 24: Midtown Nursing Home

Midtown Nursing Home, a well-financed facility, evolved a plan to expand its comprehensive chronic care program knowing that although it had a good reputation for institutional care it was not viewed by the community as a provider of home-delivered services. Its good reputation would serve the institution well in developing an enlarged program, but the institution would have to undertake new staffing, training, information systems, and marketing activities.

Midtown learned that an existing and respected care coordination/home health agency, Geriatric Services, Inc., was in financial distress that had resulted from reimbursement problems and underfinancing, not lack of quality service. Geriatric Services, Inc., had a good staff and well-designed program but could not continue under the prevailing circumstances.

A joint venture was arranged with the idea that viability of each of the two types of service would be maintained but that Geriatric Services, Inc., would in time be abolished as an entity, with Midtown Nursing Home emerging as the sole owner of an enlarged new program.

Figure 9. Sunrise Health Care Corporation.

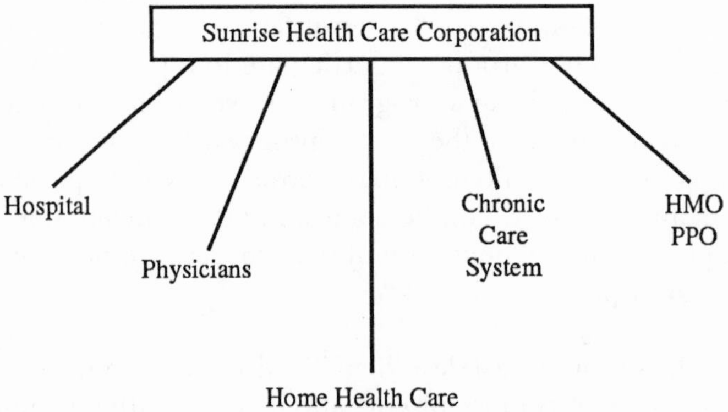

Establish a Vertically Integrated System. A third approach is the vertically integrated system within a single organizational framework. This can be best illustrated by the On Lok model (see Chapter Six), wherein one organization provides the full gamut of services under the umbrella of its ownership and administration. This structure may readily be replicated within an acute care institution that also offers chronic care services within its own organization, as illustrated in Figure 9.

Now, having taken the necessary steps to determine the most desirable organizational structure, the sponsoring group is ready to determine the financial feasibility of the proposed venture.

Chapter 8

OBTAINING FUNDS

LONG-TERM CARE IS UNDERGOING an era of unprecedented ferment and growth, simultaneously challenging the limits of public financing and regulation and providing important new market opportunities for health care providers [Hughes, 1986, p. 3].

While funding opportunities are limited, public interest in improving the availability and quality of chronic care services is increasing, especially in the area of coordination of existing resources. In this environment new opportunities have to be demonstrated through innovative use of resources, reallocation of resources, and the creation of new interests and supports.

Opportunities for financing chronic care will be organized around the following:

- Market assessment
- Expansion of the role of existing services
- Integration of services
- Capital financing
- Payment for chronic care services by:

110

Medicare
Medicaid
Private health insurance
Social Services Block Grants
Older Americans Act funds
Veterans Administration programs
U.S. Department of Housing and Urban Development programs
Grants
Waivers

Market Assessment

Income to support new programs and the interest of the public in paying for services depend upon the existence of a market. Proposed programs should be able to determine that there is a demand for particular services that either do not exist or that, as offered, are inadequate. Unmet demand is sure to occur as the population ages and the very old increase in numbers in an environment that has not adequately planned for its aging and disabled (Rice and Taylor, 1984). The market analysis for any proposed project should be conducted by specialists who are sensitive to the service needs within chronic care rather than by persons who look at new market opportunities without having sufficient experience in dealing with the special characteristics of the market. The product of a market assessment may be a decision regarding allocation of new financing or reallocation of existing resources.

While a market assessment alone may not create any new funding, the identification of needs may result in resources being made available. The assessment should therefore include identification of potential resources and techniques for gaining access to them.

Expansion of the Role of Existing Services

It is likely that most communities will have some chronic care services that can serve as the base for an enlarged program or be expanded into a coordinated system that takes advantage of established strengths in responding to a wider spectrum of community needs. New programs can add to resources already in place to increase the scale, improve cash flow, provide a referral source for the existing services, open new markets, and establish a leadership role in a growing field. The list below (Rice and Taylor, 1984, p. 37; reprinted with permission) suggests possible growth areas and the rationale for selection of each service offering for inclusion in a hospital's expansion plans. A similar review could be conducted of any existing programs to explore possibilities of expanding them.

Profile of Potential Service Offerings by a Hospital

Research and Education	Hospitals are finding benefits from participation in training programs for professionals in the growing field of geriatrics.
Information and Referral Services	Hospitals can promote profit-generating programs.
Healthcare Screening Clinics	Clinics provide seniors with an opportunity for diagnosis of untreated conditions and familiarity with hospital services.
Housing	Depending upon the health status and economic resources of an individual, the elderly person may require any one of a variety of housing situations, e.g., skilled nursing facilities, shared housing, board-

ing houses, and retirement communities. Hospitals are benefiting by participation in the development and management of such housing.

Health Education

Older people, like all other population segments, are demanding information and skills to participate responsibly in their own health care. Hospital-sponsored programs on such topics as self-examination, exercise, and nutrition can aid the preservation of health.

Psychological and Emotional Services

Hospitals can extend their services by offering grief resolution counseling that encompasses volunteer and "second career" opportunities and telephone reassurance ("daily call") programs.

Social Health Maintenance Organizations (S/HMOs)

A method of combining health, social, and financial resources is being experimented with as an offering to the elderly. This model of service delivery relies on voluntary enrollment and prospectively determined prepaid rates. Hospitals can serve as an investor

Diagnosis-Specific Support Groups

in the S/HMO or as a provider organization via contract. Peer level discussion groups specific to particular diagnoses, such as alcoholism, blindness, cancer, diabetes, and stroke, can support older people.

Multipurpose Senior Citizens Centers

Hospitals that sponsor facilities that enable the centralization of services to senior citizens are valued as a community resource. These centers provide "one-stop" service delivery to facilitate social, recreational, emotional, and physical needs being met.

Transportation Services

A vital service to the elderly is adequate, economical transportation. Providers benefit when their patients have the means of traveling to the site of the healthcare facility.

Finance Counseling

Patients and hospitals both gain from accurate information about and efficient use of financial resources in the planning of healthcare delivery.

Legal Services

Advice regarding wills, guardianships, and other

	legal issues is ancillary to the health of the elderly.
Outpatient Therapies	Hospitals can increase access through clinics. The elderly have special needs for dentistry, vision, hearing, and podiatry clinics.
Adult Day Care	Senior citizens who do not require 24-hour care and yet do need assistance during day hours benefit from facility-based adult day care services.
Homemaking Service	Elderly persons who need assistance with personal care in their homes benefit from homemakers making regular visits to attend to these chores.

This listing is provided to illustrate the variety of opportunities that exist to develop a plan that would enlarge the existing scope of services with the goal of ultimately creating a coordinated system of chronic care. While any one service may not in itself be profit making, or even self-supporting, developing a composite of services will add to the cash flow as well as income, reduce overhead expenses, and in the long run create economies of scale sufficient to generate a financial base that will support the chronic care program.

Integration of Services

The integration of services within an organization will bring a variety of services, some of which were identified in the preceding list, into a unified, coordinated program under a single sponsorship.

While service integration may not initially generate additional income, it can result in a cost reduction to permit the allocation of additional resources to the chronic care program. An integrated system allows the provider "to control uncertainty more effectively by making more of the key variables internal to the organization. Vertical integration is a well-established business strategy that allows internal prices and controls to be instituted over broader portions of the system" (Leutz and others, 1985). Efficiency can be improved, weaker units can be helped through difficult times by stronger units, and opportunities to substitute services to accommodate the needs of the provider as well as the recipient of services can be created.

For example, the existing nursing home may develop a cost-efficient, free-standing adult day health program. In space that is not allocated for use by the nursing home residents, the new service can be established where it can take advantage of food service, office and billing services, and other services that can be purchased by the new program on demand without creating a burden upon the nursing home. In this way the nursing home's operation can be made more efficient while offering support to a new service unit. The presence of the adult day health program can provide admissions to the home, and discharges from residential care can, if appropriate, be transferred to the day program.

Capital Financing

The sources for capital financing vary with financial conditions, government loan and insurance programs, and interest rates. The list below, adapted from a table compiled by Jennings (1982), suggests the need to explore a variety of options for capital financing.

Debt

Tax-exempt debt
State health facilities authority
Local authority

Housing development authority
Taxable debt
Section 202 (FHA)
Title III OAA
Section 232 mortgage insurance (FHA)
Section 242 mortgage insurance (FHA)
Title III OAA mortgage insurance

Equity

Contributions
Sale of stock

It should be obvious that it is not adequate to consider capital financing detached from the resources needed to fund the operating program. Every effort should be made to obtain capital financing that will minimize the burden on the operating budget or, when possible, delay repayment of capital expenditures until the initial period of program development has been achieved and a sufficient cash flow has been generated.

The opportunities for capital gifts to not-for-profit or public agencies should not be overlooked. These may be particularly attractive when a new program proposes an innovative service, responds to a pressing community need, or is of special interest to a prospective donor. A good illustration is the contribution to an Alzheimer's treatment unit made by the family of an Alzheimer's patient for whom it had been impossible to find an appropriate care facility in the community.

It is a good idea for every not-for-profit or public agency to establish a program of endowments and opportunities for giving, carefully outlined and made known to key constituencies in order to stimulate capital gift giving.

Payment for Chronic Care Services

The simple reality is that there is no single or simple way to gain access to appropriate funding for chronic care services. There are multiple sources of funding, often requiring that discrete segments of the program be aligned with funding sources directed to specific groups of persons or narrowly defined situations. An organization's exhaustive search of all the current opportunities is followed by negotiation for access to the funds. While public funding makes up a major share of the resources available for chronic care services, private funding from insurance carriers or families should not be overlooked.

The interrelationships among public funding sources and programs serving chronically ill older persons are illustrated in Figure 10.

Figure 10. Major Federal Programs Funding Community Services for the Elderly.

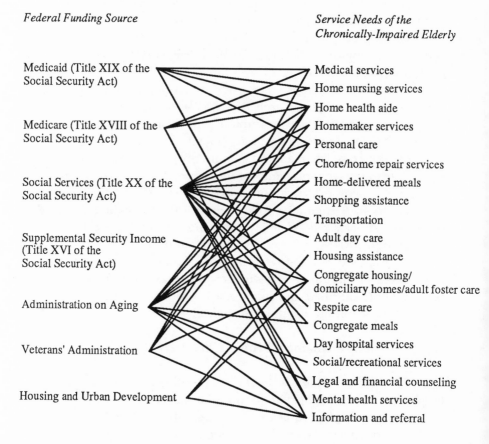

Federal Funding Source

Service Needs of the Chronically-Impaired Elderly

Medicaid (Title XIX of the Social Security Act)

Medicare (Title XVIII of the Social Security Act)

Social Services (Title XX of the Social Security Act)

Supplemental Security Income (Title XVI of the Social Security Act)

Administration on Aging

Veterans' Administration

Housing and Urban Development

Medical services
Home nursing services
Home health aide
Homemaker services
Personal care
Chore/home repair services
Home-delivered meals
Shopping assistance
Transportation
Adult day care
Housing assistance
Congregate housing/domiciliary homes/adult foster care
Respite care
Congregate meals
Day hospital services
Social/recreational services
Legal and financial counseling
Mental health services
Information and referral

Source: U.S. General Accounting Office, 1979.

The intricate web of lines relating funding source to programs should make it evident that the reality of generating sufficient funds depends upon the ability to explore and use multiple funding sources. As new funding sources are identified, in both the private and the public sectors, the list on the left side of the figure can be enlarged.

While multiple funding is a necessity, it does complicate planning and implementation of a comprehensive program, because varying eligibility requirements and different administrative entities tend to lead to fragmentation of service delivery. Figure 11 more clearly identifies possible funding sources for various programs.

It should be apparent from the information presented in Figures 10 and 11 that the recipients of services—the chronically ill person and members of that person's family—would have an inordinately difficult time understanding the many sources of funding and gaining access to assistance in obtaining payment for the multiple services that are likely to be required. The importance of the managed approach provided by the care coordination service is reinforced by the need to bring funding sources for all components of the prescribed program together into a coordinated package. Some of the funding sources may be available only for demonstration programs and, while they may be valuable to initiate a program, cannot be relied upon for ongoing support.

Somers (1985) points out that state and local governments paid a greater percentage of chronic care bills than did the federal programs and private insurance companies. (This is different from the payment distribution for acute care, which is primarily paid for by Medicare and private insurance.)

Let us now examine the various funding sources in greater detail.

Medicare. Medicare has been a disappointing resource for chronic care, for while it is a health insurance program for those over the age of 65, it adheres to an acute care rather than a chronic care model. In fact, Medicare payments in Part A focus almost exclusively on short-term acute care. The Medicare omissions have created a void that remains to be filled, although that void is the focus of current remedial efforts either to revise

Figure 11. Public Financing for Services to the Elderly.

	Federal Programs				
	Title XVIII Social Security Act (Medicare)	Title XIX Social Security Act (Medicaid)	Social Services Block Grant (Title XX)	Title III Older Americans Act (amended 1984)	Title IV Older Americans Act (amended 1984)
Estimated 1985 Funding Level	$55 billion	$17 billion[a]	$2.6 billion[b]	$760 million	$28 million
Acute-Care Services	●				
Hospice Care	●	●			
Rehabilitation	●	●			
Swing Beds	●	●			
Skilled Care	●	●			
Intermediate Care		●			
Personal Care		●			
Foster Care		▲	●		
Adult Day Care		●	●		
In-Home Nursing	●	●			
In-Home Therapy	●	●			
Home Health Aide	●	●	●	●	
Homemaker			●	●	
Chore			●	●	
Congregate Meals			●	●	

Program			
Home-Delivered Meals	●	●	
Surplus Food Distribution Program	●		
Counseling	●	●	
Protective Services	●	●	
Outreach	●		
Screening and Evaluation		●	
Health-Related Services		●	
HMO	●		
S/HMO	▲		
Multipurpose Senior Center		●	
Model Projects			●
Research on Needs			●

▲ Demonstration
● Ongoing Services

[a] Represents portion (approximately 38 percent) of Medicaid estimated to be spent on the elderly.
[b] Represents estimated funding for entire program. It is difficult to determine what percentage of this amount is used for the elderly.

Source: Jennings and Krentz, 1985.

Medicare or to devise an alternative source of insuring against the catastrophic financial burdens of chronic care.

Although posthospitalization continuing care in nursing homes may be made available under Medicare for up to 100 days, such care is usually reimbursed only for a portion of that time. Payments for skilled home health care services, on the other hand, are more readily available in Parts A and B, and payments for medical services are partially covered in Part B.

In addition to the problem of limited payment resources for chronic care, there is widespread misunderstanding among Medicare-eligible persons, who often think Medicare will cover the costs of chronic care as well as it does acute care. This misperception has caused many persons to be less concerned about obtaining alternative means of private insurance coverage, and the result is a great void in coverage for chronic care.

Some providers, especially in HMOs, have negotiated a capitated Medicare rate with the federal government. On Lok is one such care provider. By contracting to receive a fee for participation in the HMO, based on the average Medicare payment per person, it is possible to produce a program that provides greater service and/or cost savings. The Medicare funding represents a financial source with potential flexibility for resourceful use of available funds to provide a combination of acute and chronic care. (For more information on Medicare, see Appendix B.)

Medicaid. Medicaid is the primary public source of funding for chronic care, representing "about 80% of all public money spent on nursing home care. . . . About 40% of all Medicaid funds are spent on long term care" (Jazwiecki, 1984, p. 76). A major problem with Medicaid has been its requirement for "spending down," or divestiture of assets, which in effect requires families to pauperize themselves in order to gain access to this insurance program. This has especially severe consequences when the program does not permit a married couple to consider their assets separately, which would permit a spouse who does not require institutional care to maintain some degree of financial independence. Some states do permit a separation of the assets of a married couple for Medicaid eligibility; this policy should be a standard one for all states.

Continuity of care is made difficult by the separation of Medicare and Medicaid funding, although some innovative programs (for example, On Lok) have found a way to bridge the differences by bringing both sources of payment into a capitated chronic care program. The inability of an individual provider to modify the national programs does not preclude opportunities to redesign chronic care programs into a continuum of health care that minimizes the differences between acute and chronic care while demonstrating the ability to fashion a comprehensive program that has capitated funding from both Medicare and Medicaid. (For more information on Medicaid, see Appendix B.)

Private Health Insurance. Private health insurance is on the threshold of major innovations. These may take the form of indemnity policies, chronic care benefits merged with Medicare, group chronic care policies, and/or social and health maintenance organizations (Meiners and Gollub, 1985). Private insurance programs become more inviting as older people recognize the problems associated with having to spend down to qualify for Medicaid and the limitations of Medicare.

One of the most inventive approaches, which employs the idea of a prepaid, vertically integrated system of managed care, is the social HMO developed at Brandeis University's Health Policy Center. This social HMO has four essential features. "First, a sponsoring organization (or organizations) takes responsibility for integrating a wide range of acute and chronic care services into a single system. Second, this new entity serves a membership that is representative of the elderly. Most importantly, it enrolls both disabled and able-bodied elderly. Third, the S/HMO is paid on a prepaid capitation basis—by both individual members and third parties. The S/HMO pools these premiums to pay for member services. Fourth, the S/HMO is at risk for service costs. That is, the organization takes responsibility for meeting its budget, and it stands to experience some level of profit or loss for its effort'' (Greenberg, Leutz, and Wallack, 1984, p. 77).

Four sites were selected nationally to demonstrate the viability of the social HMO under the auspices of the Brandeis Health Policy Center. They are:

- Elderplan, a subsidiary of the Metropolitan Jewish Geriatric Center in Brooklyn, N.Y.
- Medicare Partners, a joint venture between the Ebenezer Society and Group Health, Inc., in Minneapolis, Minn.
- SCAN Health Plan, a subsidiary of the Senior Care Action Network of Long Beach, Calif.
- Kaiser Permanente Medical Care Program of Portland, Oreg.

Creating each social HMO model required the reorganization of existing sources and organizational plans of the sponsors. It was "not merely an extension of its current business, and the sponsoring sites realized early on that they were creating something that was likely to change them, could easily compete with them, and might eventually overwhelm them" (Greenberg, Leutz, and Wallack, 1984, p. 78). Table 6 illustrates the different sets of internal and external opportunities and constraints each sponsor had to confront.

The Brandeis demonstration social HMOs illustrate one of the new insurance opportunities. An offshoot of the concept behind them is the Life Care at Home Program, also coordinated by the Brandeis University Health Policy Center, and funded by the Robert Wood Johnson Foundation. This new program attempts to insure the older person against major health risks while concentrating on maintaining the individual's household as the primary site for the delivery of services. Institutionalization may be provided if required, but, in contrast with typical life care centers, institutionalization is not a requirement for participation in the program. (For more information on private health insurance, see Appendix B.)

Social Services Block Grants. Social Services Block Grants are federal block grant funds that are distributed to state governments and then allocated to local programs. While this money is not intended exclusively to assist the elderly, a large portion of it is made available for noninstitutional programs such as adult day care, senior centers, and services that offer homemakers, home health aides, and personal-care aides. Priorities for the allocation of these funds are established at the local and state

Table 6. Overview of Social HMO Demonstration Sites.

Site sponsors	Type of sponsor	Relationships to partner(s)	Key opportunities and obstacles
Metropolitan Jewish Geriatric Center (MJGC), Brooklyn, N.Y. (Elderplan, Inc.)	Comprehensive chronic care agency	Capitation contract and bottom-line risk sharing with small affiliated medical group. Community hospital contracted on per diem basis.	*Opportunity:* Large untapped market *Obstacles:* Creating an HMO and medical group
Kaiser Permanente Medical Care Program, Portland, Oreg. (Medicare Plus II)	Large established HMO	No partners—S/HMO added to existing Kaiser system.	*Opportunity:* Use experience and reputation *Obstacles:* Creating LTC services
Ebenezer Society, Minneapolis, Minn. (Medicare Partners)	Comprehensive chronic care agency	Partnership agreement with large established HMO for all acute medical. Bottom-line risk sharing.	*Opportunity:* Expertise and images of partners *Obstacles:* Competitive HMO market
Senior Care Action Network (SCAN), Long Beach, Calif. (SCAN Health Plan, Inc.)	Case management/ brokerage agency.	Separate contracts with established medical group and medical center hospital. Both on capitation/risk basis.	*Opportunity:* Large untapped market *Obstacles:* Management and incentives in the system

Source: Greenberg, Leutz, and Wallack, 1984. Reprinted with permission.

levels and must be in keeping with federal guidelines. This process provides opportunities for advocacy on behalf of aging services programs to identify the needs of older people and to promote the importance of chronic care programs.

Pima County Aging and Medical Services, for example, merges Social Services Block Grant funds with Older Americans Act funds, state funds, and county funds to provide a variety of noninstitutional services that include care coordination, adult day health, transportation, personal care, and homemaking services.

Older Americans Act Funds. The Older Americans Act established in 1965 a network of federal, state, and area agencies dedicated to serving the elderly. Funds are awarded for service, research, demonstration, and educational programs. Major recipients of funds under this act are Area Agencies on Aging and nutritional programs. During the past few years the Administration on Aging has participated in an annual consolidated Office of Human Development program that invites applicants for funding to propose programs related to a list of federal priorities. Organizations serving the elderly should obtain the announcements of this project and determine where their particular interests might coincide with this invitation for grant applications.

In the Pima County program this source of funding was obtained and the money used to demonstrate the value of support groups for families of Alzheimer's patients. As a result of this demonstration, it is expected that the county will continue to fund the staffing required to conduct the program as an ongoing service.

Veterans Administration Programs. The increasing number of male and female veterans who are reaching an advanced age has caused the Veterans Administration to intensify its activities in chronic care. Opportunities exist in many communities, especially where VA hospitals are located, to contact the local VA office to reach agreements for providing institutional and noninstitutional services for veterans.

Contract opportunities exist to provide nursing home care, adult day health services, and some home-delivered services to patients discharged from VA hospitals. The presence of a stable group of VA-supported participants may provide the core clientele that is critical to successful development of chronic care services.

U.S. Department of Housing and Urban Development Programs. The Department of Housing and Urban Development (HUD) has provided alternative opportunities for funding a variety of building programs backed by federal insurance, which results in a lower interest rate than may be available in the marketplace. HUD has also provided congregate services moneys for persons living in subsidized public housing and offers some resources for research and demonstration projects that may be useful in developing and testing new service opportunities.

The HUD Section 202/8 program to provide low-cost housing for the elderly offers a combination of low interest rates and rent supplements for projects that serve elderly and handicapped persons whose income is below the federal guideline. This program, which has been the source of many new housing programs for the elderly, also provides rent subsidies for elderly persons living in housing *not* supported under Section 202.

Grants. Grants may be available from public or private sources either to implement an agenda for the funding agency or to respond directly to a proposal for a demonstration of an innovative approach. To be innovative a program need not be esoteric; it may simply bring together some existing components of the caring system in a new configuration designed to improve quality of service, reach out to an underserved population, or reduce the cost of providing service. There are directories of foundations that identify areas of special interest, and these should be reviewed as a guide to potential resources.

Waivers. Waivers of Medicare or Medicaid regulations permit a modification of the policies related to public funding in order to demonstrate a cost-saving approach or a change that will enhance the coordination of services into a continuum of care. But use of waivers need not be restricted solely to these purposes. Waivers are used for merging funds in the On Lok program, for example, as well as in the demonstration social HMOs.

Although the funding of the chronic care continuum remains a major obstacle, it is not an impossible hurdle to overcome. The evidence of accomplishments of the programs cited in this book illustrates how innovative programs have been able to attract funds from a variety of sources and merge them into a comprehensive program. The growing recognition of the importance of coordinated chronic care systems provides the background against which new and innovative programs will be assessed. The money is there, but it must be pursued with the assiduity of a prospector—also in search of gold—using the tools of planning, searching, and creativity.

Chapter 9

DESIGNING ENVIRONMENTS FOR THE ELDERLY

WHEN SOCIETY FINALLY OVERCOMES its ambivalence about the value of life for the ill elderly, then and only then, can we be assured of a positive environment in long term care facilities [Miller, 1982, p. 77].

Environments determine the expression of emotion and behavior. One is involuntarily quiet and in wonder on the first visit to the nursery after a baby is born. Even though excited, one whispers in the tense excitement of a close tennis match or is silently moved at a beautiful symphony. But shouting and jumping to one's feet are the natural way to express one's feelings at a boxing match or football game.

Environments give us all kinds of clues to expected behavior. The atmosphere of a church or art museum sets the stage for a spiritual experience. Rolling green lawns invite barefoot exploration, and tumbling ocean waves tempt us to a cooling dip. Darkening skies and lightning can evoke a sense of danger and responses varying from defiant shouts to quiet tension.

Traditional health care environments tend to cause us to be quiet and to stand in awe of the white or scrub-green uniforms and the sophisticated technology, both of which represent a higher authority.

When older people are part of the environment, their presence sometimes creates negative responses from others: objections to a new retirement center in the midst of family residences, physical harassment of a feeble elderly woman, rejection of the frail and forgetful, revulsion at signs of our own mortality, withholding of professional skills and competencies because of an uncertain life span. On the other hand, there may be reverence and respect for the aged, or greater helping and caring.

The environment of an older person influences that person's self-image, responses to other people and the community, and capacity to continue to live and thrive and love. The absence of evidence of caring on the part of others—certainly a component of the environment—can be as unyielding to the older person as the barriers to freedom of movement that stairs impose on someone in a wheelchair.

Furthermore, the importance of environment increases with the dependency of the individual. The more feeble a person becomes, the less ability that person has to control the environment and the more important the environment therefore becomes—as ally or adversary. There is no doubt that developers of chronic care services possess the power to influence the environment they create and to make that environment responsive to those who will live there. This is true not only when the development involves new facilities but also when, for example, all or part of an existing facility, such as a hospital, is to be retrofitted as a service center for the elderly, or individual residences are to be modified to make them more responsive to the changing needs of older persons.

Health care providers should be familiar with critical design features for the elderly so they can transmit their expectations to architects and other designers. Just as health care administrators need not be accountants but must be able to read and interpret accounting reports, such administrators must understand environmental issues that affect the elderly to see that they are appropriately incorporated in the setting of any chronic care program.

This chapter is intended to help developers of chronic care programs become more sophisticated contractors of environmental design services. One of the major concerns is for accessibility, or "the ability to circulate without hindrance within the microenvironment; the freedom to perform daily living activities; the right and the means to maintain privacy; the knowledge that the user is in control, requiring minimum outside assistance" (Raschko, 1982, p. 2).

If in fact the design is good for the elderly, it will be equally supportive to others who use it, because it will be comfortable and take little time and energy to maintain. The environment should, to the greatest degree possible, be responsive to behavior and physical needs and do all it can to ensure that disabilities do not become handicaps.

Especially in relation to housing arrangements for the elderly, the specific areas that should be carefully evaluated and perhaps modified are entries to the home or apartment, the kitchen and eating areas, and bathrooms. Accessibility to all of these is particularly important.

The goal is to develop environments that fit the user, support expected behaviors, and do not intrude. A successful environment is either unnoticeable or delightful. If it is to serve the needs of the elderly, it should do the following:

- Include features that reflect understanding of the aging process
- Be compatible with changes in perceptual and/or physical capabilities
- Be barrier-free to persons in wheelchairs or handicapped
- Support recovery, retention, and development of abilities rather than disabilities
- Be flexible in response to changing interests, life-styles, expansion of services, and improved methods of service delivery and/or systems

General Design Criteria for the Elderly

A Minneapolis architect who specializes in designing environments for the elderly, Jack Bowersox, has established certain design criteria, outlined below, that take into consideration the sensory losses experienced by older persons (Bowersox, 1984).

Vision. As the eye ages, the lens hardens and yellows. The hardening of the lens, which occurs unevenly, will cause bright rays of light or glare to be misdirected within the eye and impair vision. This vision impairment also occurs when an older person is sitting in direct sunlight. The pupil dilation and contraction rate is slowed, which impairs vision when the field of vision changes from dark to light areas. Older persons require more light than younger people to accomplish a task without eyestrain. Design responses are:

- Glossy or shiny surfaces should be totally avoided due to reflective qualities that cause glare. Surfaces of special concern are floors, walls, tables, countertops, and cabinets.
- Light fixtures are the main source of glare. Fixtures that conceal the source of light, such as wall-mounted valance lighting, should be selected.
- Exterior lighting should be located in a manner that prevents it from shining into windows.
- Although colors are an effective means of communicating with older persons, the yellowing of the lens causes difficulty in distinguishing blues, greens, and pastel colors. Very dark navy, black, brown, and gray tones are also difficult to discriminate. Bright colors may be read clearly as contrasts on neutral backgrounds. Reds, oranges, bright blues, strong greens, and violets should be used. Bold patterns, such as stripes, should be used instead of small contrasting, intricate patterns that may cause dizziness.

Hearing. Older persons experience difficulties in discriminating normal conversation against the background of compelling noises that may be generated by the building's mechanical systems, traffic (inside and outside the facility), echoes, music, clatter of dishes, and other conversations. As hearing loss begins to occur, high frequencies will not be perceived. Design responses are:

- Partitions with a high sound rating should be used around noise-generating areas such as mechanical rooms, maintenance rooms, kitchens, shops, laundry rooms, music rooms, and activity rooms.
- Sound-absorbing materials should be used on vertical and horizontal surfaces. These materials include acoustical ceilings, carpeting, wall coverings, draperies, and wall hangings.
- Decorative acoustical baffles can be hung from the ceiling to reduce echoes.

Touch. The sense of touch becomes increasingly important with the years, in that this sense is not reduced as a mere function of age. As other senses diminish, the older person will rely more on a sense of touch to pick up stimuli from the environment. Design responses are:

- Wall surfaces may be effectively covered with materials having tactile distinctiveness.
- The substitution of wood for metal is not only more visually attractive and characteristic of a residential setting but also warmer and more inviting to touch.
- The use of Braille in the chronic care environment is of little use to most older persons. Because they have encountered vision problems at an advanced age, Braille has not and probably will not be learned. Raised or recessed letters and numbers should be used, however.
- Decorations having tactile interest or function, such as draperies, coarse wall hangings, plants, and nonabsorbent upholstery, should be provided.

Orientation to Time and Place. As short- and long-term memory losses begin to occur (often accelerated by relocation trauma), orientation to time and place becomes increasingly difficult—and increasingly important. Numerous and repetitious environmental clues will reinforce the cognitive mapping process. Elements that can be changed for various seasons should be designed into the environment. Clocks and calendars should be prominently located. Special daily events should be posted and highlighted. Design responses are:

- Clocks with nonreflective faces that indicate time in large Arabic numbers should be located at eye level.
- Environmental clues should be provided through the use of signs. Graphic signs using simple letter styles (with small or no serifs) should be located no higher than four feet from the floor. The letters should be recessed or raised one-eighth inch and be a minimum of one inch tall for readability through touch.
- Wherever possible, symbols that are culturally familiar, such as a barber pole outside the barber shop, should replace signs.

Personalization. Each individual, old or young, has the need to impose his or her personality on the environment. This may take the form of remodeling and/or decorating a house or apartment upon occupancy. Once this has been accomplished, the environment can usually be considered "home." Older persons who have been separated from family and friends are often especially attached to their personal furniture and household belongings. The environment should be designed to allow opportunities for older residents to use pieces of their own furniture and to display personal effects and pictures. Design responses in the institutional environment are:

- Use of the resident's own bedspread should be encouraged.
- Large areas should be provided in resident rooms for pictures and other wall hangings. This can be accomplished through the use of such wall coverings as cork.
- Personal decoration should be allowed in the hallways at entry doors. This will help in orientation and in reducing the institutional feeling.

- Residents should be encouraged to hang their own pictures in shared areas of the facility and to place their own furniture in lounges.

Mobility and Agility. The aging process generally has its most *see*noticeable effect on the individual's mobility and agility. Arthritis and muscular complications diminish finger dexterity, making various controls and latches hard to manipulate. Limits of reach become restricted between knee and shoulder height, and walking may require assistance from canes, walkers, and wheelchairs. The head movement necessary for looking from left to right or for looking up to the ceiling may become restricted. Leg movement may be limited, making it difficult to climb stairs or enter a bathtub. General mobility throughout the environment becomes increasingly more difficult. Activities of daily living become more time-consuming or, in some cases, even impossible.

Every effort should be made to create environments for older people that are as adaptable as possible to their individual levels of mobility and agility. Design responses are:

- Avoid using benches or couches for seating. Chairs with arms and backs should be provided.
- Provide hand rails with a flat area on top where the forearm can be rested, but narrow and equipped with recesses for finger grip. Two mounting heights should be considered: one for upright, ambulant individuals who use their forearms for support (mounting height at three feet, six inches) and the other for wheelchair users who use the rail to pull themselves down the hall (mounting height at two feet, six inches).
- Because the highest percentage of accidents occur in the bathroom, this space must be carefully analyzed for functional and safety considerations. The base floor should be large enough to accommodate wheelchair users. The toilet should be of standard height, with an elongated bowl on a recessed base, and preferably wall-hung. This type of bowl will provide clearer access by providing more free area for wheelchair foot pedals. If a toilet set higher than standard

height is required, a filler piece can be added beneath the seat to achieve any desired height. Various types of grab bars may be attached to the toilet seat, eliminating the need for blocking the walls. This approach will also allow for simple modifications when a resident's mobility level changes.

- The sink should be mounted on a countertop to allow for wheelchair access. The drain should be located to the rear of the fixture to allow a greater maneuvering area for someone in a seated position. A single, elongated lever should be used for water control. Mounting location should be to the side of the sink in the direction of the toilet, to eliminate the need to reach and stretch to the rear of the fixture and also to provide access for someone sitting on the toilet.

- Mirrors should be located on the wall beside the sink. This will allow the nearsighted user who is not wearing corrective glasses to get close to it without leaning over the sink when shaving or applying makeup. This is especially important to a wheelchair user, as is having the mirror low enough to reflect the image of someone seated.

- Medicine cabinets should be provided in side walls to eliminate the need for reaching over the countertop.

- The shower should provide for wheelchair access (no curb), and the floor should have a nonslip surface. Nonslip surfaces should also be used throughout the toilet and bathing areas. A horizontal grab bar should be mounted on the walls of the shower at a three-foot height. A vertical grab bar should be mounted adjacent to the shower head and water control. A telephone-style "portable" shower head should be provided, along with a single-lever water control that contains a nonscalding mixing valve. A swing-down seat should be provided in the shower area within reach of the shower head and control valve. A shower curtain and rod should be used, rather than a sliding door.

Design Suggestions for Specialized Programs

Consistent with the orientation that individuals using care services will each be uniquely different from everyone else and that unique and special needs justify specialization of programs, buildings used in care programs must also be designed to respond to different needs and to specialized programs. Especially germane are design issues related to the development of a building-oriented program such as a nursing home, congregate housing facility, or adult day health center.

If programs are to respond to the unique needs of individual users, the buildings in which the services are provided must support this approach. It follows therefore that all buildings in which chronic care services are provided will not be of the same design.

Nursing Homes. Nursing homes have typically been designed with anchor points at nurses' stations and corridors leading from these stations to patients' rooms (see Figure 12).

The design is often predicated on the orientation of the site or the availability of some standard nursing home floor plan. The designs presented in the diagram are frequently defended as desirable because they permit a view of the entire floor of the nursing home from the nurses' station.

Several counterarguments to this logical explanation are possible, however.

1. Nursing staff do not perform their services by viewing the population.
2. Nursing staff are generally not seated at a fixed location observing the corridors.
3. Observing corridors does not permit determination of what is happening in any of the bedrooms or public rooms.

What is required is a design that is responsive to a program and population. Some questions to be asked are:

1. What are the needs of the population being served in the particular facility or section of a facility?
2. How can nursing staff be assisted in serving this population through the design of the building?
3. How can staff other than nurses be supported in their functions by the building design?
4. What needs other than nursing care should be addressed in the building design?

Figure 12. Typical Nursing Home Design.

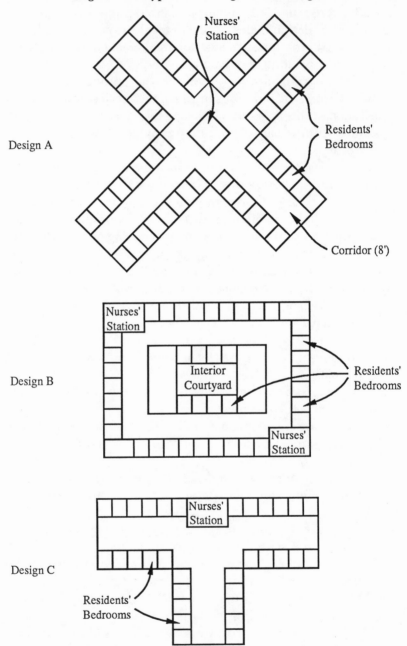

While these questions are generic to any area of the build-ing, they become more critical as special needs of a portion of the population are identified. For example, decisions regarding the necessary proximity of staff to residents differ considerably for residents who are bedbound and those who might wander away from the facility and require special protection without restricting their mobility or constraining them to a bedroom.

In facilities designed for the care of residents who need careful monitoring, it is critical that nursing services be organized to permit quick response and frequent observation. Any building with corridors will have nurses' stations at some distance from many of the rooms. Positioning of nurses' stations and related services at the ends of corridors makes it necessary for staff to make frequent trips from their stations to residents' rooms. Ideally, the design for providing intensive nursing home ser-vices to residents requiring frequent monitoring (those, for ex-ample, who are respirator-dependent or are receiving parenteral/enteral therapy) would place nursing staff equidistant from most of the residents' rooms at a central location where observation is convenient.

The ideal physical arrangement would be a circular build-ing with the nurses' station at the center, with a clear view of all rooms. Glass walls for the rooms, which can be curtained for privacy, would permit maximum visibility and access to any room. The number of rooms in the circle would determine the diameter of the circle and the distance between the residents' rooms and the nurses' station. Depending upon design con-siderations, the circle should be changed to a square or an elongated rectangle, maintaining some of the benefits of the cir-cular design although sacrificing some observation opportunities and equal proximity to all rooms. (See Figure 13.)

In designing environments for residents who are severely demented, it is important to minimize opportunities for disorien-tation. It can be confusing for such a person, uncertain where corridors lead, to step out of a bedroom and be faced with a decision whether to turn right or left. Confusion can be reduced if, instead of facing a corridor, the bedroom door opens onto a large social area where people and activities can be readily seen.

Figure 13. Circular or Rectangular Nursing Home Floor Plan.

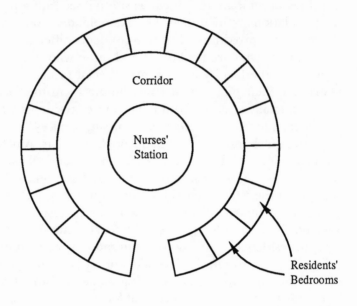

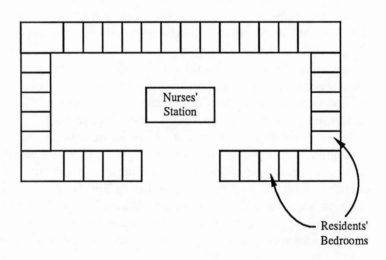

Here the individual can respond to a source of music or other diversion, possibly the aromas of a meal being served. (See Figure 14.)

Figure 14. Floor Plan That Reduces Confusion.

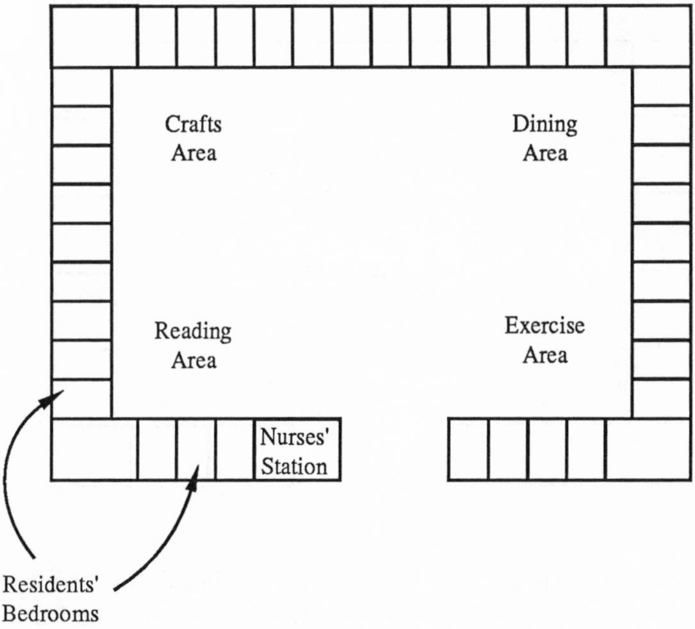

Crafts Area

Dining Area

Reading Area

Exercise Area

Nurses' Station

Residents' Bedrooms

If the primary focus of the program is to be personal care, the priorities shift to more privacy for residents, less surveillance by staff, and additional spaces for social activities. In this situation the nursing service area can be less accessible, as shown in Figure 15.

While considerable attention has been given to location of the nurses' station in recent years from the point of view of design and while the location and services to be provided at the station are often defined by nursing home codes, careful consideration should also be given to making certain there is adequate contact between nurses and those receiving services. This im-

Figure 15. Floor Plan for Personal-Care Facility.

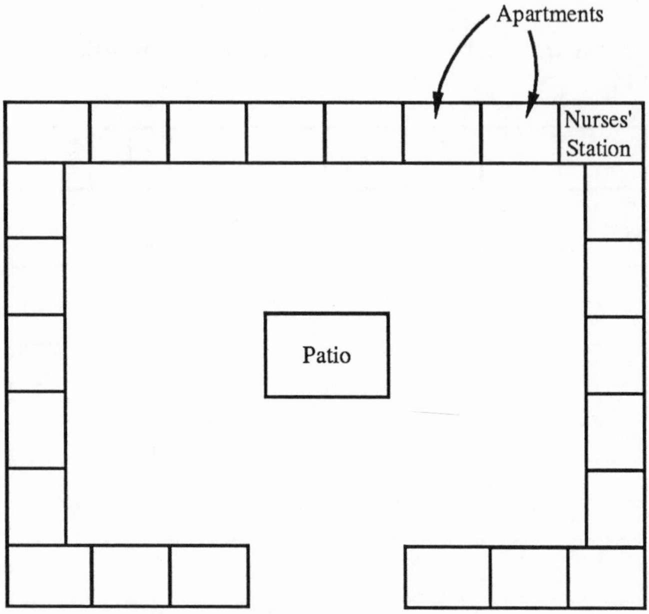

portant issue supports the argument for smaller living and work units, which can be achieved in even a very large institution by creating modules that respond to different resident groups. Differentiated modules can also be adapted from one use to another in response to changing service needs over time.

It is increasingly apparent that nursing home care will in the future be targeted to specific populations, and that flexibility in changing to respond to changing needs will be increasingly important. The module concept offers:

1. The ability to respond to the needs of specific target populations that require specialized services.
2. Positive orientation to ensure that adequate nursing services are available.

3.   Flexibility to change program orientation with changing needs.

The nursing home that is responsive to these goals is conceptualized in Figure 16.

Issues in the design of nursing care units are of special concern to hospitals that are attempting to convert all or a part of their buildings to nursing home care. Frequently the buildings being converted are old ones, whose design features the central nurses' station from which corridors emanate to the patients' rooms. Some buildings may have toilets and bathing facilities in central locations rather than in individual patient rooms.

Some multistoried buildings may not be protected by fire sprinklers and may have limited outdoor recreation areas. Although serviceable, such buildings may have to be retrofitted to serve a population or program different from that for which it was designed.

Two important design concepts are pertinent to developing a new facility or retrofitting existing buildings. The first is that facility design should not encourage residents' greater dependency or appear more institutionalized than is consistent with the level of care provided. For example, an environment supporting independent residents should not look like a nursing home by having clearly visible such characteristics as call lights, nurses' stations, and medical equipment. This is particularly important when a hospital building is converted to a residential facility. In such cases considerable effort may be necessary to conceal features that clearly identify the previous use; attention must be paid to the size of the rooms and the relationship of rooms to other services, and to providing areas for privacy and access to the out-of-doors.

"It just doesn't look like a residence," may be the response to a retrofitted hospital even after substantial efforts have been made to effect cosmetic changes. Sensitivity to this dilemma may, depending on the design of the hospital, discourage use of a building as a residential environment or create a real challenge to designers asked to minimize the adverse institutional appearance.

Figure 16. Conceptual Design of a Modular Nursing Home.

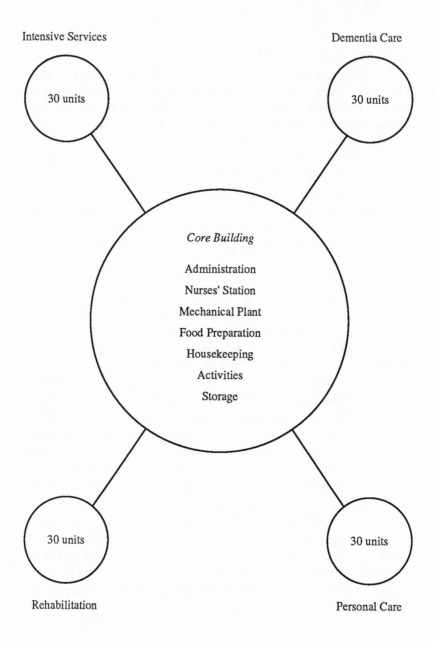

Intensive Services

Dementia Care

30 units

30 units

Core Building

Administration
Nurses' Station
Mechanical Plant
Food Preparation
Housekeeping
Activities
Storage

30 units

30 units

Rehabilitation

Personal Care

The second concept, stressed by Lawton (1974), is known as environmental press. It says that the more disabled the population using a facility, the more critical the design, because disabled persons are so dependent upon the supports of the environment to achieve the highest possible level of independent functioning. Environmental obstacles that might go unnoticed by a fully ambulatory individual may loom as major obstructions that prevent full participation in a desired activity by someone who has a severe physical limitation.

A person in a wheelchair may not be capable of manipulating the chair over even a minimal threshold or up or down a steeply sloped corridor. A person who has had cataracts removed and wears contact lens implants may be temporarily immobilized by the glare of sunlight, poor lighting, or a reflection from a shiny floor surface. Similarly, a person with senile hearing changes may be overwhelmed by broadcast music, usual institutional noises, and reverberation of sound from institutional surfaces.

Another area of concern is the institutional environment's ability to enhance residents' orientation by reducing to a minimum factors that might be confusing. This is particularly true for persons who have difficulty in being cognizant of time and place. It has already been noted that long corridors having transitional points that require decisions about which way to turn may be bewildering and may cause the resident to avoid the encounter and become dependent on others to assist in finding the way.

Because this type of confusion may result in an undesirable expenditure of staff time, the person may be placed in a wheelchair to speed up transfer, or may be served meals in the bedroom to save time and trouble. Such alternatives discourage independent ambulation and socialization on the part of the resident, certainly not a desirable outcome.

Placing electrical outlets higher than usual or installing plumbing handles that are easily turned may seem small details, but they are important to achieving the desired outcome of maximum independence.

Hospitals usually are built vertically, and when it comes

to a point of redesign for chronic care, every effort is likely to be made to retain street-level areas for reception, administration, recreation areas, and other areas that display the mission of the institution. Equally important is the need to retain street-level space for the care of demented persons, so that they can have access to outdoor areas where they can wander but still be safe. The presence of such a unit on the street level may, however, cause concern about the public image of the facility, if visitors and newcomers immediately come in contact with the unit providing care for demented persons.

In redesigned hospitals a central institutional dining area is generally housed in what was the hospital cafeteria. Such an arrangement is not the most desirable, because of the noise and confusion it generates as well as its unsuitability to meeting the needs of persons having varying requirements for assistance and attention. It would be more desirable to locate small dining areas adjacent to living spaces, thereby bringing together people who have similar service needs. Dining then can be a more intimate and sociable experience.

A frequent design-related concern of developers of a nursing home is site selection. Where should a nursing home be located? A good site for a nursing home is in a residential area near a hospital and physicians' offices. Other important considerations are:

- Availability of fire and police protection
- Proper zoning
- Utilities
- Public transportation
- Suitable topography
- Absence of noise or safety hazards
- Adequate size to provide for outdoor recreational areas and future expansion

A nursing home must conform to a number of codes and regulations, many of which affect design. These include:

- Local and/or state building and fire codes
- State Health Department regulations

- Federal regulations for nursing homes
- National Fire Protection Association Life Safety Code

Congregate Housing. At the other end of the care-level spectrum is congregate housing, an institutional environment designed specifically to maintain independence.

Site selection for congregate housing facilities involves the same criteria listed for nursing homes, except that proximity to a hospital and physicians' offices is not a priority.

Very minimal staff support is provided, but security is available around the clock. Central facilities for meals and recreational activities are provided, although the apartments are generally equipped with kitchen facilities and full bath.

In these environments, personal privacy for each apartment is essential, as is limiting the horizontal distance between apartments and central facilities so residents can easily move about without assistance.

To reiterate, no one standard plan can serve all the requirements of the different levels of housing and institutional programs for the elderly in the best possible way. Every building design must be compatible with the goals and intentions of a particular program so staff members can direct their energies to serving residents rather than overcoming the building's deficits.

Furthermore, the design of a building should take into consideration the future needs of the population so that, if necessary, changes can be made to respond to "aging in place." After an extended period of time, residents often experience increased dependency as a result of having become older. Their changed health care needs may preclude their remaining in the environment that previously was suitable.

The developer of congregate housing needs to consider whether the planned environment can meet the expected needs of a population that has aged in place. One solution is to design a series of areas that individually meet a progression of care requirements, making it possible for a resident to transfer from one area to another that is more appropriate.

While it is not easy to predict future needs accurately, it is important to provide multiple options for building use by accommodating possible changes in the future. This may involve the ability to relocate partitions, add electronic equipment, or introduce care centers in areas initially designated for alternative uses. If the need for future changes can be anticipated, appropriate preparations for possible modifications can be made, providing flexibility rather than commitment to a predetermined plan. The necessary modifications can be completed at minimum cost if advance planning provides for options by identifying central points that permit changes in plumbing and electrical or electronic systems.

Adult Day Health Care. As noted earlier, there may be different populations that can be served by adult day health programs, and it is necessary to decide what group is to be accommodated in order to determine an appropriate design. Adult day health services generally attract people who are frail; large numbers of them are demented and will require close supervision. Some of the same design characteristics described in the discussion of nursing home design are also suitable for this type of program—for example, the use of open spaces that permit ease of supervision and the provision of protected outdoor areas where those who might wander will be safe. There should be quiet spaces for resting or napping as well as for small-group interactions.

In addition to toilets there should be a bathing area, preferably with a stable lift attachment in a tub, as well as a washing machine and dryer to respond to problems of incontinence.

Because meals will be served, a serving kitchen is required even if food is not prepared at the site.

Designing to Meet Needs of Staff and Families

While much of the focus of design strategies is on the needs of residents, it should be noted that any building should also respond to the needs of staff and residents' families. The building should support staff members and enable them to implement the mission of the organization. Staff should feel an alliance with the building and know that it permits full utilization of personnel energies to provide quality service.

Especially now that nursing homes are expected to provide services requiring electronic technology, constant monitoring, and specialized breathing and feeding devices, it is important to have these kinds of equipment readily accessible as well as having patient rooms positioned for frequent observation and monitoring of the status of residents. The appropriate design for units where this kind of high-technology care is administered is comparable to that of a hospital intensive care unit.

Staff quarters, places where staff can retreat for relaxation or meals, should provide a comfortable setting out of visual contact with the persons being served. The space, its decor, and its furnishings should communicate an appreciation for the value of staff and staff members' importance in carrying out the mission of the organization. Providing care for persons with debilitating chronic illness can be very demanding, and every effort should be made to reduce the pressures during periods of relaxation.

On-site day care services for young children of staff members can be a valuable employee benefit, feasible when the employees are sufficiently numerous to support such a program. If the chronic care institution is near other health facilities, as when an old hospital adjacent to a new acute care building is converted to chronic care, inviting others to share the child-care program can broaden the market.

Family members may want to use some quiet indoor space other than the bedroom (especially if the bedroom is shared with another resident) when they visit a relative. Some outdoor visiting spaces may also be desirable. Opportunities for dining with relatives provide ways to celebrate special occasions and holidays and should be made part of the design and be readily available to family members.

Much has been learned about architectural and decorating techniques that help overcome physical or sensory limitations. Careful attention to creating an environment that fosters independence and self-confidence is itself a therapeutic measure. Also important is recognition that when an institution becomes a person's home, it should be as homelike as possible.

Chapter 10

IMPLEMENTING A
COORDINATED CARE SYSTEM

MANY ANALYSTS HAVE SUGGESTED that the effectiveness of public dollars for long-term care could be maximized if existing fragmented public funding streams were pooled to finance a coordinated array of long-term care services [Hughes, 1986, p. 221].

Implementing strategies are what make a program happen when the decision to proceed has been made and a program has been selected. The essential steps to be taken include the following:

Determine financial resources
Develop an implementation plan
Involve the Area Agency on Aging
Integrate medical and social care organizations
Orient personnel to a new field
Conform to licensing requirements
Meet with community groups of older persons

Determine Financial Resources

It is critical at the outset of implementation that accurate estimates be prepared and funding sources be assured. While the preparation of operating budgets and specification of the details of financing will occur after the program has been described and costs have been identified, it is important to know that moneys to operate the program will be available. These will include funds to support the planning activities, the start-up costs, and the ongoing costs of providing the services.

Although payment for services by third-party payers may be a significant resource, venture capital will have to come from other sources, such as reserves, endowments, or investments. Grant funds may also be available to initiate and demonstrate the value of a new and innovative program. Continued support from some grant sources is often available.

Costs will be incurred in many areas, some of which are identified below.

Planning Costs. There will be expenditures necessary to plan and develop the project and establish it as a functioning entity. These up-front costs are burdensome at the outset, but they should be recovered through program-generated income. Although money for comprehensive planning and for financial and market analysis may be hard to come up with, it represents an investment that should not be avoided.

Start-Up Costs. Adequate initial operating funds must be provided at the start of any program, and for some time thereafter it is likely that there will be few participants; yet the entire program must be made available, offering services of the highest quality and in the full amount required by each individual. This means that staffing the project for what later will be a large client group will increase start-up costs. Careful budgeting is required to project these costs, and financing must be adequate to assure that all services are functional.

Lack of sufficient start-up funds may result in the failure of a well-conceived project, as illustrated in the following case study.

Case Study 25: Start-Up Problems at Mission Plaza

A proposal to develop Mission Plaza Retirement Community appeared to be based on a well-considered concept, and the project was thought to be properly financed. However, at the conclusion of negotiations with the financing institution, the reserve set aside for operations during a two-year start-up period had been converted to a mortgage reserve, and this money was no longer available to meet operating costs. The bank had never before financed a congregate housing program and thus had qualms regarding the protection of its investment. It did not understand the cash requirements during rent-up (that is, the time period before substantial occupancy is achieved) and the adverse impact on marketing of elimination or reduction of operating reserves.

The developers were ready to break ground and did not want to resume a search for financing for the project. They had erred in not ensuring the availability of sufficient start-up operating funds. Their plan, market study, contractor, and interim and permanent financing proved insufficient to guarantee the successful implementation of the project. What should have been a twelve-month rent-up period had to be extended to twenty-four months because of the lack of marketing and early operational funds, and as a consequence there was a substantial loss of income. Word circulated throughout the community about the project's slowness in paying vendors, and many prospective tenants were reluctant to move into an unstable setting.

Operating Costs. The operating budget will reflect the ongoing stable costs for operation based on known sources of income and expenses at optimal occupancy. These should be projected over a five-year period and take into consideration anticipated cost adjustments resulting from inflation, salary increases, and other changes in either income or expenses. It is useful to project best-case and worst-case alternatives for start-up and operating budgets to help management establish sensitivity to change and to learn to recognize trends that may require modification in the budget.

Opportunity Costs. Any estimates of income and expenses should take into consideration the "opportunity costs" associated with increased utilization of a variety of services or reutilization of space or services that might otherwise be unused or nonproductive of income. For example, the chronic care program may ensure higher utilization of a sponsoring hospital, or the enrollment of a large group of older persons in a program may have an impact on economies of scale.

Conversely, the planning and preparation of the new chronic care program may demand administrative time that should be allocated (and budgeted) to the development of the new program.

Develop an Implementation Plan

Program implementation can be staged by decision points representing critical junctures in the process. For example, obtaining funding and gaining access to the funds are critical milestones. Additionally, obtaining appropriate licensing or authorization determines the ability to advance to the next stage, as does the commitment of personnel essential to the program. Developing legal documents, contracts, operating manuals, and a marketing plan are additional key decision activities. A sample format for scheduling an implementation plan is shown in Exhibit 1.

Involve the Area Agency on Aging

Chronic care programs can benefit greatly from association with various components of a well-established aging network, particularly the Area Agencies on Aging. Every community in every state is served by an Area Agency on Aging, an essential part of the aging network established by the Older Americans Act of 1965. This federal legislation created the Administration on Aging within the U.S. Department of Health and Human Services as the national focal point of services to the elderly, to encourage the development of programs to assist the elderly by providing grants to local communities from the Department of Health and Human Services.

**Exhibit 1. Implementation
Plan for Adult Day Health Care.**

	Months Scheduled for Completion									
	1	2	3	4	5	6	7	8	9	10 →
Mission and Market	→									
Organizational Plan	→									
Pro-Forma Budgets	→									
Financing	→									
Site Location	→									
Licensing and Certification	→									
Staff Recruitment	→									
Staff Employment	→									
Furnishings	→									
Transportation	→									
Management Plan	→									
Marketing	→									

It is important to note that a recent revision of the Older Americans Act specifies that the Area Agency on Aging should be involved in "services designed to assist the older individual in avoiding institutionalization and to assist older individuals in long term care institutions who are able to return to the communities, including client assessment through case management and integration and coordination of community services such as pre-institution evaluation and screening and home health services, homemaker services, shopping services, escort services, reader services, and letter-writing services, through resource development and management to assist such individuals to live independently in a home environment" (Older Americans Act, 1984 Amendments). Area agencies are also expected to concern themselves with prevention of abuse of older persons, to use the resources of an ombudsman at the state level to act on complaints by older individuals who are residents of chronic care facilities, and to advocate for the well-being of such individuals. The area agencies in many communities have been instrumental in the development of new services for the elderly. The coordinator of chronic care services in any community would be well advised to consult with the local area agency to determine how those services could contribute to the existing complex of services, supplementing established efforts but not duplicating programs already in place. A solid relationship with the area agency can be a valuable asset. The absence of such a relationship may place the new program in conflict with other providers of chronic health care services.

The new arrival to the scene of chronic care may also find that many community agencies offer care coordination services with which the area agency probably is familiar. It would be prudent to explore the possibilities of integrating such efforts into the chronic care system rather than setting up what may be a duplicative service. For example, in the Pima County Long Term Care System, care coordination is a communitywide function assigned to three well-established community counseling agencies. The county's chronic care program has signed contracts with the sponsors of these three agencies to provide their services in specific geographic areas of the county. The long-term care system thus has access to the professional expertise of experienced and trusted organizations, and the agencies share a caseload rather than feeling threatened by a competitive, possibly duplicative newcomer in their field. The agencies can be objective for the client, because they are not representing a referral source, the source of payment, or the service network implementing the plan of action they recommend.

Meeting frequently with friends in the health and social services, with area agency personnel, and with other groups serving the elderly will be helpful in establishing and maintaining good communication and working relationships. It would be wise to make a list of all the community's service agencies, to identify those involved in any aspect of the chronic care system, and to determine how plans can be made to integrate those that should become part of a coordinated program.

Of course, there are communities or agencies that may choose to develop a free-standing, vertically integrated program within their own organization. The decision to proceed in this mode should not be made until the option to coordinate with existing entities has been explored and deemed inappropriate to meet the sponsoring organization's goals.

Integrate Medical and Social Care Organizations

Historically in the evolution of chronic care systems, there has been a schism between the medical care and social care organizations. The new sponsor of a chronic care system often demonstrates a specialization in or a predilection for either the medical or the social aspects of care; there is a strong tendency to build the program around the area of greatest familiarity. Chronic care systems must find a way to merge the medical and social care systems. It is essential for the leadership of a chronic care system to work closely with both types of professionals and establish alliances across disciplines to make possible service that can occur only when people of different disciplines combine their expertise in new and innovative ways. The developing chronic care system cannot be expected to have all the skills and resources required within its own structure, so it must reach out for available community resources.

For programs having an orientation that is primarily social (for example, Area Agencies on Aging, counseling agencies, and similar groups), it will be necessary to incorporate a strong health and medical care component. This can be achieved through affiliation with a hospital, group of medical care providers, HMO, or other medical practice group. Conversely, when the initiating organization has a medical care orientation, it will be wise for the group to reach out to one of the social care organizations in its community or to add this essential care component to its program. In order to be truly comprehensive, a chronic care program must be responsive to the multiple health care needs of the chronically ill person, and also to that person's family and social network. Where the person lives and how he or she obtains nourishment, manages housekeeping, and participates in recreational activities are as significant to the maintenance of a quality life-style as gaining access to competent medical care.

What is unique to the comprehensive chronic care organization is its ability to merge what historically have been the disparate characteristics of two separate systems.

St. Vincent's program, profiled in Chapter Six, is a good example. This program, which is part of a large metropolitan hospital, is physician-directed, but its focus is primarily upon enabling each of its clients to continue to live at home by ensuring access to a coordinated medical and social caring network. Physicians write the orders, but decisions are made by a care team whose members interact to design the most appropriate care plan for the individual client. The living arrangement and personal-care services delivered in the home supplement medical care and permit a person who otherwise could not remain at home to go on living there comfortably and securely.

Orient Personnel to a New Field

We can gain a better understanding of chronic care systems by examining the environment, rules, associations, and participants involved. Those who have backgrounds in health-related professions can benefit especially from an effort to look for commonalities between acute and chronic care fields and to make transitional leaps from familiar territory to the less familiar setting.

As one such transitional leap, if I were preparing to develop a chronic care program I would probably want to join a trade or professional association. (Trade associations differ from professional organizations in that the latter may, in addition to the benefits provided by a trade association, assume gate-keeping responsibilities—defining standards and specifying qualifications necessary to enter the field. Items such as professional education, certification, ethics, and competency may appear on the agenda for meetings of a professional association.)

Participation in a trade or professional association is important, because it will introduce me to my peers and their values. The educational programs of the association will identify training needs of care providers and help me learn to identify the skills that are necessary for quality performance in this field. In addition, participation in a local association will put me in touch with existing chronic care services within the community, enabling me to build on and coordinate with resources already available. Attendance at annual meetings and reading association newsletters will acquaint me with public policy issues, advocacy proposals, shortcomings of existing programs, and predictions concerning emerging issues. The environment of health care is frequently reported, defined, or directed by the relevant association. The importance of such associations to health care providers is evident in the number of associations that exist and the large number of persons who participate in their meetings.

In some areas of health care, the choice of associations with which to affiliate may be clear, perhaps dictated by professional standards. For example, the hospital administrator may belong to the American Hospital Association and the American College of Healthcare Executives. The same administrator may also belong to the American Medical Association (if a physician) or to the American Nurses' Association (if a nurse). If the hospital has a religious affiliation, there may be additional identification with and participation in organizations of that religious group.

There is no single, all-encompassing trade and professional association in chronic health care. Rather, there are a variety of associations for which qualifications for membership are determined by employment, education, and organizational affiliations; those of greatest interest to chronic care administrators are listed: One unit of the American Hospital Association serves primarily as a trade association for hospital-based chronic care programs and nursing homes. The American Health Care Association and the American Association of Homes for the Aging are both trade associations primarily for institutional chronic care programs, while the National Association for Home Care responds to the interests of organizations providing home-delivered services. There are associations for adult day care, housing for the elderly, and senior centers; these are affiliates of the National Council on Aging. The National Hospice Organization is one of several groups representing hospice programs, and the National Association for Senior Living Industries represents proprietary developments in housing for the elderly. All of these groups, along with others not named, have an interest in coordinated chronic care, but none can be viewed as the primary organization representing that field. (A list of associations having activities related to the welfare of the elderly appears in Appendix A.)

The question remains: with whom does a person who is responsible for managing a coordinated chronic care organization affiliate? "All of the above" might be an appropriate answer, because each of the service areas represented by these groups is a major component of the chronic care system.

Until a specialized association is developed, it would be appropriate for a coordinated chronic care program to affiliate with a hospital association, a home care association, and an association representing institutional care. However, since most of the people who require chronic care services are old, it is essential also to establish affiliations with some of the age-related groups. While there are many such groups, especially at the state level, there are many national organizations that should be mentioned. These are the Gerontological Society of America, the American Society on Aging, the American Geriatrics Society, and the National Council on Aging. Each of these groups publishes periodicals, as do some of the trade associations previously mentioned. Many of the groups listed in Appendix A publish journals and other printed materials that respond to the interests of providers of chronic care services.

In addition to the elderly-oriented groups, there are groups interested in the issues of chronic illness for other age categories and for specific problems, including problems of the developmentally disabled, the chronically mentally ill, and chronically ill children and youth.

The presence of each of these very significant groups gives evidence of national interest in and concern for the problems of those with chronic illness. The multiplicity of the groups, and the absence of any coordinating council that brings together their disparate interests, illustrates the current state of chronic care delivery systems, which need to be brought together into a coordinated continuum of service groups. Each of the organizations listed in Appendix A is involved in chronic care and may have local as well as national activities. The members of each of these fraternal groups naturally feel a sense of ownership in some particular segment of chronic care. To fail to involve any of the interest groups in a coordinated chronic care program would be folly.

Chronic care professional and trade associations have a distinct opportunity within the dynamic environment that exists today to establish standards of performance and expectations of ethical practice that will become the firm underpinning of this critically important segment of health care in the United States.

Meanwhile, the need for an association for chronic care continues to exist; it might develop as an outgrowth of one of the existing organizations, take shape as a consortium of hospital, home care, and nursing home care associations, or adopt a new format not yet developed. The ability to achieve this goal will depend on advocacy by those who believe in the coordinated system of chronic care and on the readiness of appropriate national organizations that focus on home care, hospital care, or institutional care to undertake this role. Whatever its origins, the trade association for chronic care should represent all providers of services, whether they be located in hospitals, nursing homes, housing developments, or home care programs, and regardless of the age or infirmities of the clients served. The continued absence of a coordinating peer group will inhibit the development of essential intergroup relationships.

The models of coordinated care systems presented in Chapter Six have many affiliations, as is illustrated by the following list.

- *On Lok Senior Health Services.* National Council on Aging, National Institute on Adult Day Care (NIAD), California Association of Adult Day Services, American Health Care Association, California Association for Health Services at Home, American Association of Homes for the Aging, and California Association of Homes for the Aging. Individual staff members hold personal memberships in a number of other organizations.
- *Pima County Aging and Medical Services.* The agency is a member of the American Society on Aging and the Arizona Association of Nonprofit Nursing Homes.

- *St. Vincent's Hospital and Medical Center of New York.* The hospital's chronic care program holds no association memberships, but individual staff members hold personal memberships in a number of organizations.
- *Mount Zion Hospital/San Francisco Institute on Aging.* American Hospital Association, Association of Western Hospitals, California Association of Home Health Agencies, and California Association of Adult Day Care Centers.

Conform to Licensing Requirements

The problems that result from the lack of a coordinated chronic care system are equally apparent in the issue of licensing of chronic care organizations. Each segment of the chronic care system that is subject to licensing requirements must conform to a different set of rules and expectations, and sometimes must respond to different staff persons and offices within the licensing bureaucracy. Such a situation can only impede the development of a coordinated system, and until changes are made to rationalize licensing procedures, separate licensing will be required for hospitals, for nursing homes within hospitals, for free-standing nursing homes, and for home health care agencies. In some communities, hospices and adult day health programs also have to be licensed, again by a separate segment of the bureaucracy. Ideally, a coordinated chronic care program would be licensed as such, with licensing that included all of the services within the integrated program. For example, four of the case models we have been looking at hold the following separate licenses:

- *On Lok Senior Health Services.* California Adult Day Health Center (three licenses for three separate locations), California Community Clinic, California Home Health Agency, and California Health Care Service Plan. Although no license is required for congregate housing, city building and health codes are, as required, observed by the agency, and as a HUD 202 and 8 it must adhere to these guidelines.
- *Pima County Aging and Medical Services.* The county holds a skilled nursing facility license for the nursing home it owns

and contracts only with other facilities that hold an appropriate license.

- *St. Vincent's Hospital and Medical Center of New York.* New York
  Hospital, New York Short Term Home Care, New York
  Long Term Home Care (Medicaid required), and Psychiatric
  Day Care.
- *Mount Zion Hospital/San Francisco Institute on Aging.* Califor-
  nia Hospital, California Home Health Care, California
  Adult Day Care, California Acute Rehabilitation, and Cali-
  fornia Skilled Nursing Care.

In addition to the license requirements for the practice
of medicine, nursing, pharmacy, social work, physical therapy,
occupational therapy, and so on, the only license requirement
for administrators occurs for nursing home administrators. This
requirement evolved with the Medicaid law and was a measure
intended to upgrade the quality of nursing home care.

Meet with Community Groups of Older Persons

An important ally and source of information and support
in any community is likely to be the older people living there, who
often may be reached through such organizations as senior citizen
groups. The local Area Agency on Aging should have a listing of
such groups and may in fact be affiliated with a number of them.
Feedback on program proposals from older people is important
and will provide a sensitivity to the marketability of the product
as well as insight into the needs of prospective users.

More than any other segment of the community, older
persons themselves will be the ultimate judges of the value and
responsiveness of any program, so the developer of a coordinated
chronic care system should try from the outset to capture the
involvement of the elderly population. By meeting several representative groups from this population, identifying for them the
goals of the proposed program, and regularly seeking their
counsel as plans are evolved, an ongoing relationship with the
target audience can be established early. Maintaining a regular
and consistent schedule of meetings will help demonstrate the

sincerity of the developer's desire to receive constructive comments, even when they are critical. The value of this group process will be enhanced if the older persons consulted are made to feel that their participation has value to the program and that it has contributed to a system that is responsive to the needs of its users. Participating in strengthening their community's health care services can be a rewarding experience.

The successful involvement of community persons is illustrated below.

Case Study 26: Westwood Retirement Community

The developer of Westwood Retirement Community recognized that constructing congregate housing for older persons in the midst of a residential neighborhood would raise the ire of some residents and thereby create problems for his program. On the other hand, there was every reason to believe that the older people who would live in the retirement community would want to be part of just such a residential neighborhood. The location was appropriate, but objections could be anticipated because of the proposed change in land use for the area.

Mr. G., the developer, elected to minimize potential problems by creating a neighborhood advisory committee at the time the project was introduced to the community. A special effort was made to enlist participation on the committee by long-time older residents, and the commmittee met on a regular basis to receive comments about many aspects of the program.

The neighbors expressed greatest concern and were most involved in making suggestions about the exterior appearance of the building, building height and orientation, ingress and egress for the site, traffic generation, and the population targeted for marketing.

Mr. G. showed good faith with the neighbors by making changes to please them, at times at considerable expense to the project, which was ultimately improved through this process. When final presentation was made before the local planning and zoning commission, the neighbors were in attendance to urge approval.

A systematic approach to the development of a coordinated chronic care program should be determined and then implemented. There are some unique characteristics of agencies that serve the elderly, resulting from the passage of the Older Americans Act in 1965. Interaction with these service agencies, their trade associations, and professional groups cannot be overlooked by the new developer of chronic care services.

Chapter 11

ESSENTIALS OF
EFFECTIVE OPERATION

MEASUREMENT IS ESSENTIAL to good geriatric care. It is a crucial consideration for those developing, promoting, or practicing this still embryonic specialization. Any strategy for altering the health status of the elderly requires a technology for first assessing that health status and then detecting increments of progress [Kane and Kane, 1981, p. 1].

In this chapter the core contents of a coordinated chronic care system are detailed. Included in the core of the program—those things that are central to the development of any system, without regard to its setting or sponsorship—are the elements of controlled access, assessment, and care coordination. The characteristics to be described can be universally applied to chronic care, and reaching an understanding of them should be of equal value to the experienced practitioner of health care and to the newcomer to health care delivery.

Essential to helping the public understand and determine what constitutes appropriate service is selection of a title that correctly presents that service, a title that accurately conveys what that service does. Programs of housing for the elderly that provide such services as meals, security, recreation, and transportation are usually called congregate housing. Yet new developers, in an effort to present their facilities in the most attractive manner, have adopted other designations for such housing. Other new programs, responding to increased awareness of the incidence of Alzheimer's disease and AIDS, give the names of those ailments to services they offer, which should be done only if a program can assure the presence of a widely agreed-upon level of service and competence. Merely serving persons who have a disease should not qualify the program as specializing in its treatment.

In like manner, it is important that when the concepts of controlled access, assessment, and care coordination are used, they have a common, agreed-upon meaning and application by all practitioners.

Service to a client begins with informing the individual and the persons concerned for that individual's well-being about services available in the community, a function usually called information and referral. If a true continuum of chronic care exists, referral to it can set in motion a process through which the client is evaluated and provided the proper mix of services over time.

The three essential components of a chronic care continuum are inseparable and can be viewed as a triangulation of three processes that are mutually interdependent and supportive of one another. They are not intended to function independently. All three components should come into the process when any one is considered. The application of this process on behalf of any client should result in the most appropriate assignment of services and resources available within the context of any program or community.

Controlled Access

Controlled access, sometimes referred to as the single point of entry, serves to direct the client to the appropriate level of care or the appropriate provider of service. The person who is not knowledgeable about the full array of services available for a particular problem needs guidance to reach the appropriate service. Persons in need may reach out to a service because of its prominence or because acquaintances have used it. Selecting an agency or service in this manner would be somewhat like wearing a pair of corrective glasses prescribed for a neighbor because they were helpful to the neighbor's vision. Because of the complexity of chronic illnesses, there may be a combination of services that would be more helpful than one or another service alone.

Controlled access is also important because it requires that a plan of service be based on an assessment, which assists in determining an appropriate array of services. Managed entry into the chronic care system is intended to prevent both overservice and underservice.

In order for the controlled access concept to be effective, especially in the broker model (see Chapter Four), it is critical that the organizational interests of participating groups be recognized. These participants are expected to give up some portion of their autonomy, so they are entitled to have a reciprocal relationship by which they gain access to clients, are rewarded for participating in a quality program of respected reputation, and benefit from the advantages of a large-scale organization. Benefits may include increased referrals and utilization of services, enhancement of educational opportunities for employees, and greater organizational stability.

Assessment

Rubenstein (1983, 1984) suggests that assessment can circumvent inappropriate use of health care services, prevent waste of scarce resources, and contribute to avoidance of imposed disability resulting from inappropriate diagnosis and labeling of older persons. For example, persons who have been labeled as senile may very well be written off for any physical rehabilitation, even though they may have capacities that could be nurtured through caring programs. Rubenstein also hypothesizes that successful assessment programs will lead to improved diagnostic accuracy, more appropriate placement of persons in the health care system, less dependency on skilled nursing facilities, improved functional status of the elderly, and more appropriate use of medications.

Research results that confirm all these anticipated benefits of assessments are not available, but considerable anecdotal evidence provides substantial support for the belief in the value of assessment to the provision of a comprehensive care plan and improvement of the quality of services to the elderly client (Applegate and others, 1983; Moore and others, 1984; Rubenstein, Rhee, and Kane, 1982).

Critical to assessment in chronic care is the paradigm that examines what Katz and Akpom (1976) refer to as activities of daily living—the assessment of functional capacities that typically include bathing, dressing, transferring, toileting, and feeding. These in fact are performance measures that determine capacity for independence and identify areas of dependency that, if appropriately ameliorated, will increase independent functioning. In addition, the individual's cognitive capacities, social interactions and family supports, eating practices, resources in the physical environment, and mental health functioning are generally included in assessment methodologies.

Individual assessment that leads to care plans characterized by achievable goals helps the care provider become sensitive to the need of the person receiving care to perceive progress toward those goals. As a challenge to the self-fulfilling prophecy that chronic care implies decline and the uselessness of intervention, the appropriate use of assessment can identify strengths as well as weaknesses and contribute to the improvement of function and status as opposed to merely witnessing decline.

Assessment becomes a tool for encouraging maintenance of wellness and identification of resources within the individual, the family, and the environment that can contribute to the wellness of the individual. Wellness is not only the absence of pathology; it is also maintenance or improvement of functioning. The increasingly frail individual is highly vulnerable to adverse changes in the environment, so the available resources of the family, home, social network, formal care system, and access to transportation become important components of both the assessment and the care plan. Wellness of the individual can be enhanced by increased resourcefulness in using the environment to compensate for lost functional capacities.

Assessment becomes an important resource to family members as well, helping them to understand the value and significance of the environment to the maintenance of wellness for their relative and giving them goals for improvement and a work plan that defines realistic expectations for family participation in care. Of particular importance is helping family members to be objective, which in turn can lead to increased competence and confidence in their ability to participate effectively in the provision of chronic care. Family participation can have great impact both on the quality of life for the older person and on demands for public expenditures for chronic care.

Kane and Kane (1981) provide a thorough discussion of assessing the elderly and of the uses of measurements in chronic care, as well as a review of multidimensional measurements, the assessment instruments commonly used today. They also urge increased use of systematic measurement, avoidance of casual diagnostic labels, and the need for methodological research into how the measures perform and what they measure.

Baker (1980), who reviewed fourteen assessment instruments, notes that the proliferation of such instruments and the difficulty in developing a single assessment methodology is understandable in the absence of clearly delineated treatment or care programs and the difficulty of translating assessment findings into care plans. In contrast to acute care, chronic care of the aged shifts from a focus on disease or pathology to a focus on function, and then from function to intervention. Each of these transitions increases exponentially the factors to be considered in a comprehensive assessment, which is further complicated by the many possible variations in intervention. When an individual's limited economic status, constrained public funding, or a limited array of chronic care services available in a community restrict intervention, the significance of a detailed, often costly, assessment may be questioned.

Unless the assessment results in improved comprehensive

services, it is legitimate to ask whether assessment has any impact on the provision of services. It is especially important, however, to maintain the assessment function when constraints of limited funding or service options exist, in order to identify the need for additional services or for more public support of chronic care programs. In addition to being important to the individual being assessed, assessment contributes in a significant way to the accumulation of data, which are an essential planning resource that can influence the availability of chronic care services and access to them.

The care coordinator typically coordinates the assessment process, making assignments for specific services on the basis of needs presented by the candidate. The care coordinator, often a person who has a social work or nursing background, involves other key persons in the assessment team to supplement his or her own expertise. In addition to social work and nursing personnel, the team should include a physician and a rehabilitation specialist.

The assessment may be accompanied by a medical evaluation, drug inventory, or financial statement, depending upon the program for which the individual is being assessed. Lawton (1976) created a hierarchy into which the levels of competence determined through assessment could be placed to describe accurately both the abilities and disabilities of a particular individual.

The overall goal, according to Baker (1980), is to develop a multipurpose approach and methodology to rationalize clinical and planning-level decision making and resource allocation. This goal can be achieved through the use of a comprehensive assessment instrument and by matching the results with an inventory of services and resources available in the community.

One illustration of the application of these principles into a functional system can be seen in the Geriatric Functional Rating Scale of Grauer and Birnbom (1975), adapted in Table 7. A second illustration is the assessment instrument used by the Pima County program, a copy of which is attached as Appendix C.

Table 7. Geriatric Functional Rating Scale.

		Observation	Score
1.	*Physical Condition*		
	A. Eyesight	Good	0
		Watches TV	
		Reads	
		Does needlework	
		Distinguishes faces	− 3
		Sees light only	− 10
	B. Hearing	Good	0
		Hears loud voices	− 3
		Deaf	− 5
	C. Mobility	Is fully mobile	0
		Dresses	
		Carries parcels	
		Rides bus	
		Uses cane, or should use one	− 3
		Is dependent on railings	
		Requires use of cane and other support	− 15
	D. Pulmocardiovascular function	No restrictions	0
		One flight of stairs	− 3
		One city block	
		Partly or totally bedridden	− 20
	E. Diet	No restrictions	
		Restricted	− 3
2.	*Mental Condition*		
	A. Disorientation	None	0
		Time	− 3
		Person and/or place	− 15
	B. Delusions	None	0
		Mild-severe suspiciousness	− 3
		Overt	− 10
	C. Memory Loss	None	0
		Benign	− 3
		Malignant	− 20
	D. Energy and Drive	Normal	0
		Hypoactive or hyperactive	− 5
	E. Judgment	Intact	0
		Impaired	− 5
	F. Hallucinations	None	0
		Auditory and/or visual	− 10
3.	*Functional Abilities*		
	A. Reads and writes letters		+ 2

B. Uses telephone   + 5
C. Banks and shops   + 5
D. Prepares simple meals and bakes   + 7
E. Washes, dresses, and toilets self without assistance   + 5
F. Uses public transportation   + 7
G. Is able to take own medication and follow diet   + 10

4. *Support from the Community*

A. Enjoys ethnic compatibility   + 2
B. If living alone, gets support from reliable relative,
    friend, neighbor, janitor   + 10
C. Is able to shop at reliable grocery (one willing to
    deliver when necessary)   + 5
D. Available supportive and recreational facilities:
        Clubs geared to aged   + 2
        Church, synagogue   + 1
        Library   + 1
        Park, shopping center, restaurant, movies   + 1
E. Geographic availability of:
        Public health nurses   + 2
        Meals-on-Wheels service   + 2
        Homemaker services   + 2
        Friendly visitors   + 2
        Hospital with emergency and clinic facilities   + 2
        Public transportation   + 2

5. *Living Quarters*

Has elevator service or lives on ground floor   + 3

6. *Relatives and Friends*

A. Is not married but lives with compatible and helpful
    relative or friend   + 5
B. Lives with incompatible relative, friend, or spouse   0
C. Lives with able and compatible spouse   + 10

7. *Financial Situation*

A. Totally independent   + 5
B. Dependent on helpful relative   + 3
C. Dependent mainly on pension and/or community
    resources   0

                                        Total plus score   ____
                                        Total minus score ____
                                             Final score   ____

Source: Adapted from Grauer and Birnbom, 1975.

Kane and Kane (1981) note that in this rating scale, professional judgment is needed to rate the physical and mental
condition of a client, and that items on the community support

issues are of particular interest. For example, points are awarded for the ethnic compatibility of a person within the neighborhood, availability of delivery services from local shops, and the availability of various recreational opportunities and health and social services.

The Grauer and Birnbom approach is particularly interesting because it diverges from most standard assessment instruments as it seeks to determine the availability of supports that will help the individual maintain independence. "If such an approach could be refined and proved reliable and valid, then one could try systematically to alter the outcome by changing the predictors, arranging for stores to deliver, providing a janitor who can be called in emergencies, adding recreational and other services, and so forth" (Kane and Kane, 1981, p. 263). In many ways this assessment instrument goes to the heart of the chronic care system and requires an understanding of the impact of environment on the individual.

Another instrument suggested for determining the ability of an individual to perform the activities of daily living is the HRCA Vulnerability Index (Exhibit 2), developed by the Hebrew Rehabilitation Center for the Aged, which asks the following questions:

Exhibit 2. HRCA Vulnerability Index.

1. Now I will ask you about your meals. Do you prepare them yourself?

    ____ Yes   ____ No

If yes, ask: Do you have great difficulty doing it yourself?
If no, ask: Do you need this help?

    ____ Yes (P)   ____ No

2. Do you take out the garbage yourself?

    ____ Yes   ____ No

If yes, ask: Do you have great difficulty doing it yourself?
If no, ask: Do you need this help?

    ____ Yes (P)   ____ No

3. Are you healthy enough to do the ordinary work around the house without help?

    ____ Yes   ____ No (P)

4. Are you healthy enough to walk up and down stairs without help?

    _____ Yes   _____ No

5. Do you use a walker or four-pronged cane at least some of the time to get around?

    _____ Yes   _____ No

6. Do you use a wheelchair at least some of the time to get around?

    _____ Yes   _____ No

7. Could you please tell me what year it is?

    _____ Correct   _____ Incorrect

A. *Record number of (P) boxes checked for Q. 1-7*

A. _____

8. In the last month, how many days a week have you usually gone out of the house or building in which you live?

    _____ Two or more days a week
    _____ One day a week or less (P)

9. Are you able to dress yourself (including shoes and socks) without help?

    _____ Yes   _____ No (P)

10. How much of the time does bad health, sickness, or pain stop you from doing things you would like to be doing?

    _____ Seldom, sometimes, or never
    _____ Frequently or most of the time (P)

B. *Record number of (P) boxes checked for Q. 9-11*

B. _____

C. *Person is functionally vulnerable if*

"A" box greater than 1 or
"A" box = 1 and "B" box greater than 0
check (   )
if vulnerable

C. _____

Source: Morris, Sherwood, and Mor, 1984. Reprinted with permission.

Kane and Kane (1981) provide a summary of the requirements for measurement used in an assessment instrument. These requirements are shown in Figure 17.

Figure 17. Schematic Presentation of Criteria for Assessment Instrument.

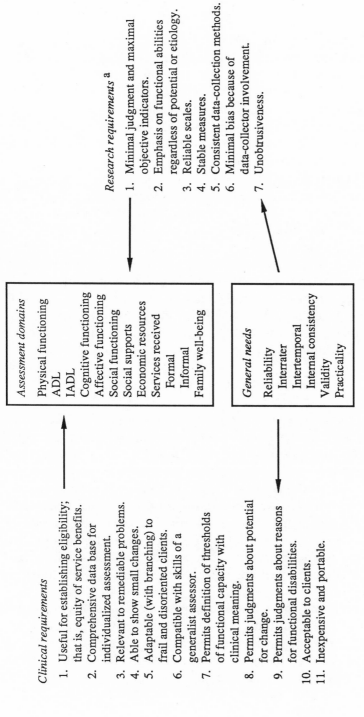

Assessment domains

Physical functioning
ADL
IADL
Cognitive functioning
Affective functioning
Social functioning
Social supports
Economic resources
Services received
Formal
Informal
Family well-being

Research requirements [a]

1. Minimal judgment and maximal objective indicators.
2. Emphasis on functional abilities regardless of potential or etiology.
3. Reliable scales.
4. Stable measures.
5. Consistent data-collection methods.
6. Minimal bias because of data-collector involvement.
7. Unobtrusiveness.

General needs

Reliability
Interrater
Intertemporal
Internal consistency
Validity
Practicality

Clinical requirements

1. Useful for establishing eligibility; that is, equity of service benefits.
2. Comprehensive data base for individualized assessment.
3. Relevant to remediable problems.
4. Able to show small changes.
5. Adaptable (with branching) to frail and disoriented clients.
6. Compatible with skills of a generalist assessor.
7. Permits definition of thresholds of functional capacity with clinical meaning.
8. Permits judgments about potential for change.
9. Permits judgments about reasons for functional disabilities.
10. Acceptable to clients.
11. Inexpensive and portable.

[a] For those variables used in evaluation.

Source: Kane and Kane, 1981. Reprinted with permission.

Assessment in chronic care can provide assurance that the individual will be protected from misdiagnosis and inappropriate care and be given access to the services most responsive to his or her needs. An appropriate match of needs and services can be achieved only after a comprehensive assessment of the individual's strengths, weaknesses, and potential—an assessment that also takes into consideration the family, social network, and environment.

Furthermore, the person assessed should be a member of the assessment team, providing input and sharing in the design of the care plan. Only after the completion of the assessment, review by a multidisciplinary care planning team, and integration of the client's plans and expectations can the implementation of a comprehensive treatment program be initiated. The bridge between the assessment and implementation of the treatment program is generally referred to as case management, although, as has been explained, the term *care coordination* is preferable; it minimizes the implication that the client is the passive recipient of a managed-care program.

Care Coordination (Case Management)

Care coordination is the process of organizing and supervising the delivery of services to persons whose chronic problems require a program of care that is both comprehensive and coordinated.

It provides access to the entire service system and ensures the coordinated delivery of multiple services to individual clients. Basic to care coordination is an initial broad-based assessment of the client's needs. In addition, the care coordination process ensures that a service plan that considers all the available service solutions is written, and that the client is reexamined at intervals.

Finding appropriate resources for human services is difficult in any community. For the chronically ill person or his or her surrogate, seeking services that will respond quickly to critical living problems is at best a challenge. The effectiveness of the chronic care system in providing appropriate services at the right time is dependent upon the care coordinator. While descriptions of care coordination abound, one of the best is the following identification of the primary activities encompassed: "Case management [care coordination] refers to a system of locating, coordinating and monitoring a defined group of services for a defined group of people. The purpose of [care coordination] in continuing care is to make the use of community institutional resources more systematic. The [care coordinator] has a dual focus: on meeting the client's individual needs and on making good use of the community's resources. The components of [care coordination] include: case finding, assessment, care planning, service arrangement, monitoring, and advocacy on behalf of the client" (Kane, quoted in Evashwick, Ney, and Siemon, 1985, p. 5).

Care coordination functions are described by Callahan (1979) to include the following: making collaborative arrangements to assure continuity of services regardless of the auspices of the provider; making necessary care arrangements; referring to appropriate services and coordinating their delivery; arranging for items and services covered by insurance; maintaining a continuous relationship with the individual; acting as a service broker by matching individual needs and resources; and ensuring delivery of services.

It should be expected that care coordination will be required over a long period of time, increasing in its intensity as the client's needs increase but also diminishing when the client's needs diminish and the client and his or her social supports become able to assume greater responsibility for the management of the chronic problems.

As a result of the use of care coordination, it should be expected that the following will be accomplished:

- The quality of care will be enhanced as a result of the coordination and continuity of services.
- Persons admitted into the system will have access to all the other services available within the system.
- Clients will receive neither more nor less care than is needed but will be provided care appropriate to their needs at any

time; the care plan will be modified as required to respond
to changing needs.
- Health care resources will be allocated on the basis of clients'
  needs.
- Community resources will be used efficiently.
- The incidence of hospitalization will be reduced.

The functions of the care coordinator, while appearing
similar to those of the social worker or hospital discharge plan-
ner, should be seen as distinctly different and should be clearly
identified as a critical component of the comprehensive care
system.

Hospital social workers or discharge planners often provide care coordination for hospitalized patients, to prepare them
for leaving the hospital and to arrange for necessary continuing services. If, instead of discharge from the hospital itself, the
need for continuing care were to be chosen as the determining
factor, a continuing comprehensive care program would be offered by the hospital.

Care coordination operates as follows. The care coordinator serves a target population defined by specific characteristics. Simultaneously, the care coordinator maintains information about a variety of health, social, and support resources
within the organization and elsewhere in the community. Both
directly and using input from other professionals, the care coordinator assesses each client's social, emotional, medical, functional, and family support status, or obtains such assessment
from the assessment team. The care coordinator then prepares
a plan of care, arranging for or referring the patient to the
services needed at the time. The care coordinator may purchase services on behalf of the client or help the client find and
pay for services from personal resources or through third-party
payers.

The difficulty of locating services may be compounded
by the processes for determining eligibility for public or private
financial support and certifying an individual for a particular
service. Care coordination is necessary because so many chronically ill persons "fall between the cracks" or are ineligible for

appropriate use of existing resources. Care coordination attempts to select the most appropriate level of service for each individual and provides the transition point between the assessment process and the effective delivery of service.

Because people using chronic care services generally have multiple problems, they often find it necessary to have contact with more than one provider at a time. Care coordination relieves them of that burden. The needs of chronically ill persons are not only multiple but also continuous; so is the need for care coordination.

Advocacy on behalf of the client is an inherent part of care coordination, as the staff member seeks the appropriate service, the funds to provide the service, and assurance that the person will benefit from the service provided.

Care coordination may be needed only for certain segments of the population. Those likely to benefit most include older persons with chronic problems that significantly impair their activities of daily living, younger persons who have neurological or orthopedic impairment due to trauma, the chronically mentally ill, and the developmentally disabled.

Existing care coordination programs have generally been funded as part of demonstration or research projects, as components of state or local government screening programs, or under Title XX or the Older Americans Act. The coordinating function has to be seen as a significant part of service and as an important instrument for cost savings in chronic care. The financial viability of care coordination may be most attractive in capitated financing programs such as HMOs, where the expense of care coordination is likely to be offset by cost savings resulting from the provision of only appropriate care, and in hospitals, where early discharge may be facilitated and patient services retained within a vertically integrated chronic care system. Advocacy for the system of care coordination will be aided by the analysis of cost savings and the ability to demonstrate that the goals of improved care and control of costs can be directly attributable to the processes inherent in a comprehensive assessment and care-coordinated program.

Some communities have developed private care coordina-

tion services that function for a fee and offer services comparable
to those provided by hospitals and publicly supported community
agencies, or through demonstration grants. Hospitals, nursing
homes, HMOs, and home health agencies may choose to develop
care coordination or contract with other groups to provide this
service.

The difference between the coordinated and the noncoordinated approaches to the delivery of services is demonstrated
by the following case studies.

Case Study 27: Mrs. G—a Noncoordinated Response

Mrs. G. lived alone after the death of her husband. She
had few close friends but was very close to her daughter and
son-in-law, who visited her frequently although they lived in
another community. On one visit they found Mrs. G. depressed,
the home untidy, and the refrigerator empty.

After much reflection, the children decided that they could
not leave their mother alone and made arrangements for her
to be admitted to a local nursing home that had a vacancy.
Because they saw no need to maintain their mother's home, they
had it sold.

Fortunately, the mother responded well to the wholesome
meals, socialization, and attention she received, and gradually
her health improved to such an extent that she was able to return
home. However, since her house had been sold there was no
alternative except to rent an apartment. She adjusted well but
would have much preferred to return to her own house.

What could have happened in a coordinated controlled-
access system?

Case Study 28: Mrs. G—a Coordinated Response

When Mrs. G. was found by her children to be depressed
and apparently unable to care for herself adequately, they decided
to have her admitted to a nursing home that was part of a coordinated system of chronic care. The admitting staff there referred

the family to a care coordinator, who arranged for an evaluation of Mrs. G., reviewed the urgency of responding to the children's concerns, and conducted an evaluation of Mrs. G.'s home and social environment.

The assessment identified the depression as one that would respond to professional mental health services. The care coordinator informed Mrs. G. and her family that she had several choices. She could receive the mental health services while remaining at home, while attending an outpatient mental health day care program, or while temporarily being institutionalized for treatment. She chose to remain at home.

Meanwhile, arrangements were made for transporting Mrs. G. to a senior center, where she could participate in socializing activities and have meals in the company of other people. In addition, homemaker services were added to the service package.

Furthermore, Mrs. G.'s progress was monitored carefully to determine which services were no longer required or could be reduced in intensity, and the care coordinator kept in touch with the children to report on the progress of the care program.

The contrast between the two possible outcomes for Mrs. G. and her family makes clear the superiority of coordinated care and its greater responsiveness to a client's changing needs.

Chapter 12

INTERACTING
WITH CHRONIC CARE
CONSTITUENCIES

FOR MANAGEMENT IS THE ORGAN, the life-giving, acting, dynamic organ
of the institution it manages [Drucker, 1974, p. x].

Managerial responsibilities to chronic care programs include
aspects of management that are generic to any form of management, including health care. In addition, chronic care managers
must have a unique set of skills and must meet some special
expectations. These special expectations stem both from the need
to understand and manage programs for people who have multiple chronic illnesses and from the environment in which services are delivered.

The following list highlights some of the characteristics
that distinguish the management of a chronic care program.

- Philosophical orientation to purpose, goals, and expectations
- Patient population (the elderly) and their families
- Services provided
- Length of time services are provided

- Staffing requirements
- Sources of payment
- Amount of money available

These characteristics are translated into management expectations that require:

- Close personal contact with the patient
- Considerable involvement with family
- A prolonged period of association with the patient and family
- Frequent loss of patients by death
- Considerable involvement with community recreational, cultural, and spiritual activities
- Specialization in areas of personal care, rehabilitation, and social services
- Ability to blend the medical and social aspects of care
- Payment relationships with families, insurance companies, Medicaid, and Medicare
- Minimal and limited reimbursements for home care, institutional care, ambulatory care, and physicians' services

Unlike the administrator of a hospital acute care program, the manager of a chronic care program must maintain a personal relationship with those served if the program is to be effective. Furthermore, because the resources available for payment for services are so limited, there is certain to be concern about being able to respond to the intensity of care needs. The obvious inadequacy of resources and the potential inability to meet demonstrated needs within those resources is a constant anxiety.

- When you see a family stressed by caring for an Alzheimer's patient yet are unable to offer respite services because of lack of funds
- When you see good nursing attendants leave for better-paying positions yet cannot increase their wages due to budget constraints
- When you know how important several hours of personal

care would be in helping an individual continue to live at
home but cannot provide the service because of lack of funding
• When you know how important it would be to have an
enhanced recreation program in publicly supported congregate housing but have no funds to provide the service

Such situations give rise to concern that can readily
become an anger so acute that the administrator of a chronic
care program is prompted to leave the field.

One of the most difficult problems of hospital administrators who try to budget for chronic care services is the
need, with chronic care, to revise expectations of required staffing because of reduced availability of funds. Some hospitals,
appreciating the need to understand the different issues involved
in the environment of chronic care, contract with chronic care
administrators or chronic care organizations to administer their
chronic care facility.

Such is the case in Tucson, Arizona, where Tucson
Medical Center, a major 600-bed tertiary care hospital, operates
a new subsidiary subacute care unit on the grounds of the
hospital through a contract with a local nursing home. The nursing home administrator occupies a critical position as manager
of the program, integrating it into the local community network
and marketing its services to the community.

Figure 18 helps identify the multiple roles and expectations of administrators in chronic care and illustrates the major
constituencies that comprise chronic care services. While the
responsibilities of each of these constituencies are described in
this chapter for all aspects of chronic care, there are special
characteristics of institutional care that will be highlighted. Administration is shown as the center of the chronic care network,
surrounded by the various spheres with which it must interact.
Each of these spheres will be separately described, along with
its implications for personnel activities.

Public Officials

Many of the chronic care services, such as nursing homes,
adult day health care, and home health care, have to be licensed

Figure 18. The Chronic Care Network.

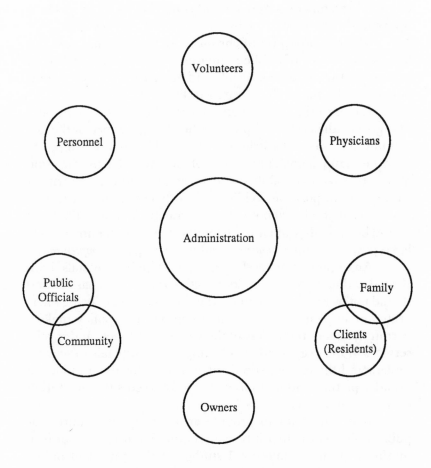

to comply with statutes at various levels of government, and their administrators must establish working relationships with public officials. Institutions that need not be licensed must be in compliance with zoning laws, building and fire codes, and health department regulations regarding food services. In addition, nursing home administrators are required to be licensed (although hospital and home health administrators currently are not). Efforts are under way to introduce voluntary certification of administrators of congregate housing programs, in order to upgrade the standard of administration of this service.

There is no aspect of chronic care services that does not have some degree of public regulation, so an understanding of how to deal with public officials and agencies is a critical component of the manager's responsibility.

It is essential to be prepared with a knowledge of the laws that govern the actions of public officials. Ignorance of the law can interfere with establishment of a working relationship. On the other hand, a good knowledge of the law and demonstration of an organization's ability and willingness to comply with it strengthens its position. While public officials or administrators of the law generally do not make the law, their actions interpret it, and because they often write regulations for enforcing it, they have power as policy *makers* in addition to policy *implementers.*

An organization's relationship with public officials, both elected and appointed, should be active rather than passive and should not be restricted to times when regulations are being interpreted or implemented. Frequent contact with policy makers permits frequent reminders of the values, successes, and special services of the organization. Inviting public officials to see and understand the organization's operation helps them to have a broader picture and to appreciate the problems the institution or service may face.

It is important to provide an educational resource for public officials, whether it be data required in preparing or promoting legislation, anecdotal studies of the impact of public policy, or simply general information. Providing quality educational experiences for public officials on a regularly scheduled basis is one way of communicating the value of chronic care.

Very often the public officials who regulate publicly financed chronic care have not previously been involved with such a program. As a result, they may have a limited perspective of the potential of the services and fail to see the real inhibitors to quality service. Putting these officials on the mailing list for all public functions of a chronic care organization will alert them to what is happening, even if they do not attend.

Community

Relationship with the community in which a service is located is especially important for institutional programs. Neighbors' concerns about traffic, trash removal, emergency services, and visitors should be openly discussed with neighborhood associations, representative neighbors, or a local focus group invited to participate in facility planning in order to make certain the institution will be viewed as enhancing the quality of the community.

Special parties or functions could be sponsored for neighbors. Elderly neighbors might be invited to holiday events, and young children might be encouraged to visit. The specific opportunities are numerous and vary according to the institution and its chosen neighborhood, but every effort should be made to avoid isolating the institution from the community.

There are ways in which serving the community can be of direct value to institutional residents as well. One home established a buddy system, matching residents with older persons living alone in the neighborhood. The resident would place a daily telephone call to his or her buddy to determine that all was going well. The community buddy would visit the home, providing friendship and companionship. The visitor would bring small items the resident needed and would share in holiday celebrations. The resident's sense of worth was enhanced by being of service through making a daily contact with a neighbor. This simple model could be enlarged or revised according to the location of an institution and its proximity to a neighborhood where many elderly persons live.

Another home, located close to an Indian reservation, broke down the barriers between the community and the tribe by inviting the Native Americans to conduct tribal rituals with members of their group who resided in the home. As a result, the tribe became comfortable with referring its members to the services provided by the home. A sensitive administration can often find such opportunities to reach out to the community and establish strong, neighborly relationships.

A special effort should be made to develop relationships with religious groups. While many institutions have chapels and visitors representing various faiths, nurturing close relationships with churches and synagogues may lead to greater parishioner interest in the institution. One church group arranged for a volunteer driver every Sunday to take a group of church members to services. The volunteers took turns providing this service, but some enjoyed it so much that they would have been happy to do it every week.

Local aging groups may also provide a resource for program development or community support and should not be overlooked as an area for administrative outreach.

Owners

Owners are a significant part of the chronic care organization, whether they be elected officials, private corporate groups, individuals, partnerships, or not-for-profit groups. Even though owners may have a great degree of responsibility for a chronic care program, they may be inadequately informed about the nature of chronic illness, the community, or the structure of community services. While owners may be responsible and competent, they may not be aware of important issues of chronic care, especially when the field is changing so rapidly. The administrator is responsible to the owner not only for management of business affairs but also for providing education to the owner regarding the community areas of service and ways to improve it, and how to provide support for employees in ways that will help them perform their functions.

Regularly scheduled meetings with owners to discuss important issues, written reports on the program's development, and circulation of pertinent journal articles help keep owners informed. Owners' attendance at conferences and workshops on issues in chronic care, as well as owners' retreats with staff and guest speakers, contribute to enriching an owner's background.

Clients (Residents)

Service to clients is the purpose of the organization and should be the force driving all activities. While the provision of direct services to members of this group will be delegated to personnel in various capacities, chronic care administrators have opportunities to establish informal relationships with the persons served. This is particularly true of institutional care, in which developing contacts with residents should be a daily concern.

Remembering that as people age they become more than ever unique, service should be tailored to each individual's characteristics and respond to them in a humane fashion. This requires that personnel get to know every client, each client's family and social network, and the client's relationship to that network. Close involvement with the client and family and the personalized approach to chronic care help chronic care providers realize the value of their services.

Continuing efforts should be made to involve residents in decisions that are meaningful to their life in the institution. Opportunities for involvement should be correlated to the physical and mental capacities of the resident, but appropriate involvement should not be neglected because *some* residents cannot participate.

And although the client and family are considered as a unit, there are also occasions when staff will approach family members separately and in a special way.

Family

Working with family members or other close social contacts is an important part of the responsibility of personnel in chronic care. Those closely associated with the client are usually involved in the provision of care and have an immediate impact on the delivery and utilization of that care. Beyond the assistance they provide—and their help should be used in a most productive way—family members also suffer trauma resulting from the chronic illness of loved ones. They therefore need caring that will help them overcome their own grief and suffering.

Family members can benefit from supportive counseling, support groups, respite services, peer contacts, monitoring of their own health, and education about the client's illness that includes appropriate suggestions for intervention. Family members may need assistance dealing with financial and legal problems, completing applications for services, or making funeral and burial arrangements. The emotional problems related to dealing with the end of the life of a loved one require especially sensitive responsiveness from providers of chronic care.

In some situations family members may indicate they need help with visiting a relative in an institution. Useful guidance on selecting an appropriate gift, the number of relatives who should visit at one time, and what to talk about can be beneficial when there is discomfort with relating to an institutional resident. Because many family members share similar discomfort at some time, some institutions support small discussion groups for family members. This service is sometimes most helpful to families of new residents, but it can be of equal value as an opportunity for ongoing dialogue regarding the issues of institutionalization.

Family members may also be involved in educational sessions that help them to understand the trajectory of their relative's incapacity and the complications of the disease involved. These sessions help to develop empathy for the person who has the problem.

Family members' comments on the quality of care a relative receives can be especially helpful. Certainly, whenever major changes in care, staffing, or patient location are anticipated, family members should be informed in advance.

Physicians

Physicians have the same responsibilities whether they care for patients in a hospital, nursing home, or office. Yet something about chronic care appears to result in diminished physician dedication. Some of the differences may reflect lower motivation when there is no possibility of cure, dwindling enthusiasm when problems must be repeatedly addressed without effecting improvement, or low financial return in comparison with that of acute care.

Some doctors are less inclined to visit patients in nursing homes or to follow up with home care; they show less commitment to nursing home patients than to hospital patients and are less responsive to the need to attend nursing home meetings or be involved in committee assignments there. Because of the minimal involvement of many physicians, nursing homes have been required by federal law to have a medical director whose function it is to be liaison between the institution and the medical community, assuring physician compliance with all aspects of care and related regulations.

With physicians necessarily becoming more involved with older people and chronic illness, their unresponsive tendencies must change; physicians need to think and act more responsibly with regard to chronic care. The providers of chronic care can help them overcome the frustrations of the field by seeking ways to involve physicians in planning for chronic care services.

Physicians may also need encouragement to participate in exciting, high-quality educational sessions, where there are opportunities to interact with skilled practitioners of chronic care. The chronic care organization can promote and sponsor these educational sessions in order to bring the latest thinking in geriatrics to local physicians.

Physicians are critical to chronic care services and new ways must be found to commit them to this practice specialty.

Volunteers

People who contribute their time to service for which they receive no remuneration can make major contributions to chronic care, especially by communicating their personal involvement and caring.

Volunteers can be used as case managers, home visitors, assistants in nursing homes and congregate facilities, friendly visitors, and professionals. Volunteers are also members of boards of directors, fund raisers, and counselors.

Whatever their role, volunteers should be as carefully selected and prepared for their work as are paid employees. Attention to them should include recruitment, screening, selection, orientation, assignment, training, evaluation, and recognition. Careful screening and assignment to jobs that are consistent with interests and skills are as critical for volunteers as for paid personnel, and great attention should be directed to making sure warmth and human concern are not made secondary to other job tasks. More than anything else, the volunteers in chronic care can provide human interaction that is motivated purely by the desire to help some other person.

While some volunteers may receive sufficient reward from being permitted to serve, it is important to others that their contribution be publicly acknowledged in some way. Annual recognition dinners, award luncheons, "volunteer of the year" selections, and recognition for years of service are some of the ways the contribution of volunteers can be publicly acknowledged. Another reward, and an important one, is being shown appreciation for their invaluable contribution by including volunteers in the organization's communication network and involving them in decision processes.

Personnel

While all of this discussion relates specifically to the many functions of administration, there are special opportunities related to the management of human resources. As in any organization, there should be formal procedures to assure that the most qualified personnel are engaged to implement the mission of the organization. These should include recruitment, screening, selection, orientation, assignment, training, evaluation, and recognition. Special attention should also be given to the importance of the interpersonal relationships that become an essential part of chronic care; in this area, role modeling by an administrator can become a standard for all employees to emulate.

Personnel should be selected for their capacity to provide personal caring, and this criterion should be included in job descriptions and taken into consideration in the amount of time designated for performing any task. Personnel should not be admonished for devoting time to caring. Rather, staff should be recognized for giving of themselves in the way they provide service—recognition that communicates the caring concern of the entire organization.

Chronic care personnel provide skilled responses to people with chronic health problems by combining technical competence with devoted caring. Chronic care differs from acute care in its focus on activities of daily living and on assisting individuals to maintain the essential attributes of their life-style, but sometimes chronic problems are exacerbated by acute episodes of illness or by complications of the chronic illness that require intervention of highly technical skills. However, cure is not always expected to be the outcome of such intervention. Instead, the result may be an accommodation to the complications of the illness—pain, limitation of mobility, reduction of activity, change in life-style, and often greater realization of the continuing chronic problems and the nearness of death. These are difficult issues with which to deal, and the provider of care to the chronically ill must have the ability to deal with them comfortably. While cure may not be in the prognosis, caring and humane responsiveness must be sustained, not reduced.

The continuity of chronicity, increased dependency, the presence of pain, and approaching death are hard for some caregivers to cope with, and many therefore avoid chronic care and seek employment in settings where the possibility of cure is an important reward for the work.

In some chronic care services all new employees are introduced to the concepts of chronic illness by experiencing what is called the empathic model. In this exercise, vision and hearing are impaired, limb movement is restricted, and other limitations are imposed; the individual is then asked to carry out a series of tasks of daily living—eating, toileting, dressing, reading, using the telephone, and so on. Some participants are placed in a wheelchair or restricted to a bed or chair in a soft restraint for an extended period of time. Participants are also shown slides that present visual loss and played tapes that simulate hearing loss.

After the experiential exercises are completed, a feedback discussion—a critical part of the training session—allows participants to share their experiences before establishing personal goals for dealing with the limitations of the persons for whom they will care.

Another important experience that can be provided to new employees is an opportunity to appreciate one another's feelings regarding the nearness of the end of life. Some individuals may discover that reflecting on their own lives as preparation for working with the dying may lead to resolution of unfinished personal business and may help them when they are needed to comfort grieving family or friends.

Oftentimes feelings related to death are expressed by clients not only in formal conversation but also through behavior and communication that may not be clearly focused. Personnel in these situations are likely to become involved, even though they are not counselors, so they need to become sensitive to the feelings being communicated.

Because these preparatory experiences, like actually caring for persons near death, make special demands and elicit strong feelings about one's own life, a channel for discussion and support should be provided.

Compensation

The reality that lower pay is often associated with chronic care services may reflect a value system that implies that curing is more highly regarded than caring. As a result, becoming a provider of chronic care is both socially and financially less attractive than working in acute care. Yet some employees may prefer chronic care, because it permits a continuing relationship with the client. Some employees may be repulsed by the technological nature of acute care and opt for the more personal and human rewards of chronic care.

Prospective employees should express a preference for employment in chronic care, based on their knowledge of that setting. Attracting personnel who have a natural affinity for chronic care can be encouraged by recognizing some of the adverse aspects of the field and making possible opportunities for relief from its burdens, especially from the repetitiveness of serving those who have chronic problems. Opportunities for respite and the availability of supportive and responsive supervision can relieve some of the tedium of this type of care.

One effective measure of relief is job rotation to different settings and kinds of care provided—from institutional care, to home care, to day health care, to congregate care. Such rotation reduces the repetitiveness of job demands and enables the employee to appreciate the extent and diversity of multiple programs and the contribution each can make to the totality of a care system.

The difficulties related to chronic care should be more widely recognized, and there should be greater appreciation of the special skills required to make the work successful. Society generally gives special recognition to those who perform important work that the majority of people are unwilling or unable to do. As the number of old and frail individuals increase, it is to be hoped that the contributions of chronic care workers will gain greater appreciation and rewards.

In summary, many constituencies comprise the network that provides chronic care. Some are more involved than others, yet all are needed to develop a comprehensive program. And at the core must be administrative leadership that provides a sense of mission and value, as well as education, to inspire everyone in the system to practice that mission in providing chronic care.

Chapter 13

PROTECTING
THE PERSONAL RIGHTS
OF THE ELDERLY

LACK OF CHOICE PRODUCES inordinately acquiescent behavior that places these elderly persons in a life situation that impairs their normal exercise of liberty. Those of us concerned with the well-being of the elderly must focus on the nature of the "liberty" to which frail, mentally impaired old people are entitled, and on the nature of developments in law, medicine, and social services, the new technologies of service delivery, and the new definitions which have been applied to those who are impaired [Cohen, 1985, p. 173].

In earlier chapters the developer of a chronic care system has been guided through an understanding of the people in need of chronic care and the system's response to their needs. In effect, the critical issues of the chronic care system have been introduced. By its very nature a chronic care service is one provided over an extended period to a population that develops an intense dependency upon the providers of care, toward which society has a decidedly ambivalent attitude. Because chronic care often results in diminution of the individual's autonomy, the developer of a service system must be alert to the significance of the dependency relationship and the potential to minimize, often unwittingly, the participant's autonomy as a competent adult in need of chronic care services.

A critical question in the provision of chronic care is whether or not by its very nature it inhibits cherished personal values and freedoms of the participants (Thomasma, 1984). Can the delivery of services to those who are chronically ill and who display considerable dependency on others for activities of daily living be accomplished in a manner that maintains or enhances the personal autonomy of the individual and family receiving care? The issue becomes more pronounced when clients suffer from dementia and cannot advocate adequately on their own behalf.

There are also legal ramifications, especially when decisions are made regarding procedures that sustain life or deliberately terminate life in an individual who is institutionalized. Do organizational imperatives take precedence over the individual's maintaining autonomy? What must the health care provider do to ensure ethical practice?

Many of the ethical issues in chronic care revolve around the theme of paternalism.

Paternalism

Those who are chronically ill, particularly the very old, may suffer breakdowns, not only of physiological functioning but also of social and personal interaction. Complicating this may be adverse reactions of society to those who are extremely dependent; those reactions may discourage the maintenance of independence and lower the self-esteem of the person being cared for (Thomasma, 1984). Whether institutionalized or receiving care at home, the individual seeking or receiving care may evoke in caregivers a strong sense of protectiveness stemming from a belief in their own superior competence to provide care and nurturing to those reaching out for help. Is this bad? That all depends.

"Paternalism is the interference with the liberty of action of an individual and is justified by reasons referring exclusively to the welfare, good, happiness, needs, interests, or values of the person being coerced. At times, however, a facade of paternalism may cover motivations which have less to do with the good of the individual than with some perception of the good of the institution, the care provider, the family, or society in general'' (Wetle, 1985, p. 259). The desire to help and the sense of self-confidence derived from the competence of the professional may, if inappropriately used, minimize the resources of the older person. The issue of paternalism is important, because it may impose activities on individuals that are not consistent with that individual's personal choice or may withhold interventions because of low expectation of response by the chronically ill older person. The potential for paternalism is heightened when the provider of care is required to act on behalf of the best interests of a client whose mental competence is impaired.

Inasmuch as there are differences in caregivers' ethical and moral values, which in turn may differ from the values of the client, it becomes critical to make responses that are biased toward the wishes of the client and to select activities that are oriented toward enhancing the personal autonomy of the client. This approach can reduce the possibility of damaging paternalistic acts. Providers of care should therefore be sensitive to the ethical and moral issues that are related to the care they give and should understand how their own behavior, as well as the implications of their decisions, will contribute to the quality of life of those they serve.

It is not sufficient for the leaders of a chronic care organization to be satisfied with their own attitudes toward paternalism, quality of life, or the autonomy of their clients. These important issues are also reflected in the beliefs and behaviors of physicians, nurses, attendants, family members, and all who contribute to the team effort of providing chronic care. An essential part of staff selection, orientation, education, and commitment must be sensitivity to the clients' needs for autonomy and a quality of life that is consistent with both the highest possible goals and the realities of situational limitations. A significant role for the organization's statement of philosophy is to communicate organizational leadership with regard to clients' rights. The philosophical orientation must then be implemented through the behavior of staff.

Clients' Bill of Rights

Organizations need assistance in identifying the ways in which they can be more responsive to individual needs. Such identification requires orientation to the special characteristics of chronic care and recognition that maintaining the individuality of each participant is possible only by avoiding a predisposition to "batch" groups of older persons who have a variety of chronic illnesses into a homogeneous group. The federal government has promulgated the requirement that all nursing homes participating in Medicare or Medicaid programs develop a residents' bill of rights. The following example illustrates the expectations of such a document.

- At the time of admission, the resident must be informed of his or her rights, of services available at the facility, and of charges for these services.
- The resident must be fully informed of his or her medical condition.
- The resident must not be transferred involuntarily except for medical reasons, nonpayment, or protection of other residents. Except in an emergency, when a nonconsensual transfer occurs, advance notice must be given.
- The resident should be encouraged to exercise his or her rights and to express grievances about the facility to staff and to outsiders. No discrimination or reprisal may occur as a result of these complaints.
- The resident must be free from mental and physical abuse and from chemical or physical restraints except as authorized by a physician or to protect the resident or other patients from injury.
- The resident must be assured confidentiality with respect to his or her personal and medical records and is empowered to authorize their release to others.
- The resident must be treated with consideration, respect, and dignity and must be accorded privacy in treatment and in care for personal needs.
- A resident cannot be required to perform services for the facility except in limited circumstances.

- The resident is authorized to associate and communicate privately with others in person or by mail.
- The resident may participate in social, religious, and community activities and, with some limitations, may retain and use personal clothing.
- The resident is authorized to meet privately with his or her spouse and, with some exceptions, to share a room with that spouse, if both are residents of the facility.
- The resident may manage his or her personal financial affairs. The facility is required to account quarterly for financial transactions made on behalf of the resident, if the facility has been authorized by the resident to handle money.

The preceding list of residents' rights applies to skilled nursing facilities; a slightly different one exists for residents of intermediate care facilities (ICFs) and for residents of ICFs for the mentally retarded. Many states have adopted their own bill of rights for nursing home residents.

While developing such a document is an important early step that will identify commitment to the autonomy of the individual receiving care, it is critical to recognize that it is only a basic statement. More important are its implementation in the training of employees and the demonstration that the care provided enhances the lives of those who receive it.

Elder Abuse

Like paternalism, overt elder abuse reflects a lack of respect for the elderly. The acts of abusers can be categorized into acts of commission (such as physically striking a patient), generally termed *elder abuse,* and acts of omission (such as not turning a patient in accordance with a prescribed regular schedule), generally termed *elder neglect* (Phillips and Rempusheski, 1986). Abuse can be communicated in the use of violent language, in the improper implementation of a care plan, or in incompetence on the part of the caregiver.

It does not matter whether the act is a purposeful one designed to cause harm or a consequence of benign neglect or oversight. Behavior may be abusive simply because of the dependency of the person receiving care, a caregiver's paternalistic attitude, or incompetence.

Sometimes the abuse is a result of frustration and despair on the part of a caregiver who is attempting to respond to the requirements of many severely ill persons; but, whatever the reason or cause, the leadership within a facility must define potential sources of abuse or neglect and take measures to eliminate them. Abuse in any form must be prevented.

Several approaches may be useful to prevent abuse. One is the careful screening and selection of employees on the basis of competence and a sense of compassion in dealing with chronic illness. At the time of employment there should be a clear communication of the program's commitment to respecting the dignity and individuality of each person who is served in the program. This philosophical commitment should be illustrated in the form of specific behavioral expectations that are reinforced by repetition, which underlines the importance of this aspect of performance.

Leaders must consistently display certain characteristics to their employees if they expect comparable performance from those employees. An effective leader must display:

- Support of the use of a bill of rights, requiring that all users of services be fully advised of their rights and opportunities
- Commitment to involvement of users in meaningful roles
- Patience in committing the time required to conduct a specific plan of service
- Careful involvement of family members
- Regard for each individual's religious, cultural, and social values
- Sensitivity to each person's needs

Providing a role model of compassion and respect for individual rights of employees reinforces the message of concern for these principles and encourages their being observed by personnel in dealing with clients. That message of concern must not be in word only, however. Advocating sensitivity to the

needs of individuals and then disciplining a housekeeper for taking time to visit with a patient is the kind of inconsistency that
must be avoided.

Compassion cannot be expected from employees who
themselves experience abuse in the form of poor staff quarters,
insensitive demands, schedules that do not provide adequate
rest, and salaries that are inappropriate for the work to be
performed.

Treating each staff member as an individual is important, because people do not react to stress in any uniform or
prescribed way. Knowing the staff and what is important to each
person, and recognizing how each reacts to the constancy of care
for the chronically ill, will make possible sensitive reactions to
signs of stress.

Stress may intrude upon the ability to relate appropriately
to the individual receiving care; how it does so will vary with
the employee. Yet there are some general signs that should alert
the administrator to investigate the extent of the potential problem. These include absenteeism, tardiness, inability to complete
tasks, frequent illness, short temper, abusive language, and
general unhappiness with the job. Any one of these symptoms
should not by itself be considered evidence of stress-related problems. Rather, it should be a warning signal, especially if the
symptom is inconsistent with earlier behavior.

Perception of a signal that an employee is experiencing
stress calls for appropriate reaction. This might be a pat on the
back and a compliment for good work, a discussion of the work
situation, a change in routine, time off, or some other encouraging response. The presence of sensitive, supportive supervisors
may be critical to personnel's well-being in stressful situations.

Enhancing the Quality of Life

The admonition to do no harm must be extended to the
use of state-of-the-art skills and knowledge to make possible the
highest level of care and caring. This includes the administration of medications and procedures such as resuscitation in a
manner consistent with a respectful attitude toward the patient.

This may also include being responsible about saying what the institution or agency can do and what it cannot. If an organization says it specializes in rehabilitation of the elderly, it should know and practice state-of-the-art rehabilitative services for the chronically ill older person. If an organization says it specializes in caring for persons suffering from dementia, it must be prepared to provide much more than good nursing care; it must be able to enhance the quality of life of the afflicted person.

One way of enhancing the quality of life for persons receiving chronic care is to give each individual the greatest possible degree of control over his or her life. This may be accomplished by allowing clients to schedule care to accord with personal preferences, to choose where and with whom to socialize, to be served food they like, and to express their individuality. This is particularly important when prolonged institutionalization is required. The milieu in which chronic care occurs, whether at home or in an institution, can be enriched by a variety of activities designed to foster individual choice and control.

Depending upon their competence, individuals may be involved in review of menus and be able to select the foods they prefer. They may be allowed to exercise choice over their leisure-time activities. A very valuable element of control is experienced when persons receiving care can be involved in selecting the persons who give care and in subsequently evaluating the caregivers' performance on the job.

Consent

One of the most significant exercises of control a client is involved in is consenting to participation in a medical or research procedure. "It is the ethical and legal responsibility of the practitioner or researcher to inform an individual about procedures, risks and benefits so that he or she can make a judgment about voluntary participation" (Tymchuk, Auslander, and Rader, 1986, p. 818).

The documents used to communicate the risks of any procedure are of great importance to the older person; they should be carefully designed to make certain they are understandable.

The small-print legal document presented under pressure for a decision may dissuade a client from expressing questions and concerns generated by the proposed procedure. Large print and simplified language on consent forms, or even a videotaped presentation, demonstrate greater sensitivity to the importance of the decision. Whenever possible, ample time should be allocated for the client to review and reconsider the content of the documents. Again, the obligation not to harm the person does not justify giving treatment over the objections of a competent person, even if it is done in the belief that the treatment will benefit the patient. Competent, informed persons have the right to decline life-sustaining interventions.

DNR and Ethics Committees. The decision not to resuscitate (DNR) is one issue that illustrates the complexity of informed consent. If the individual is not capable of directing a DNR decision, may someone do so on behalf of the patient? Even close, well-informed family members may not be able to represent the chronically ill older person. All adults are presumed to be legally competent unless declared incompetent by a court. "Only a judicial officer can declare an individual legally incompetent and appoint another person to make legally binding decisions on behalf of an apparently incompetent patient" (Nelson, 1986, p. 9).

While DNR clearly stands for "do not resuscitate," it is important to caution that it should not also be taken to mean "do not respect." Too often the person identified with the DNR receives a lower priority of treatment or is put at the end of a waiting list for care (Schiffer, 1987). DNR should not create a nonperson but rather should define the response or absence of response to a specific event. Life is no less significant because a DNR decision has been made, and the person to whom the decision applies should be treated no differently from any other patient.

The decision to resuscitate or not is not the only encounter with ethical issues related to persons near death. Individuals may choose to refuse any means of treatment or intervention. An individual who finds no value in prolonging a life overburdened with pain and disability may decide to refuse nourishment. Another may elect to be permitted to die. Such personal decisions, even when made by competent persons, may not be respected by well-meaning health care professionals who have a commitment to sustain life.

The Living Will, prepared while the individual is competent, is an instrument designed to communicate the individual's requests for treatment, in order to direct the behavior of caregivers if and when that individual becomes incompetent and is near death. Exhibit 3 illustrates the kind of language used in a Living Will.

Exhibit 3. A Living Will.

Declaration

Declaration made this _____ day of _____, 19____.

I, _____, being of sound mind, willfully and voluntarily make known my desire that my dying not be artificially prolonged under the circumstances set forth below and declare that:

If at any time I should have an incurable injury, disease or illness certified to be a terminal condition by two physicians who have personally examined me, one of whom is my attending physician, and the physicians have determined that my death will occur unless life-sustaining procedures are used and if the application of life-sustaining procedures would serve only to artificially prolong the dying process, I direct that life-sustaining procedures be withheld or withdrawn and that I be permitted to die naturally with only the administration of medication, food or fluids or the performance of medical procedures deemed necessary to provide me with comfort care.

In the absence of my ability to give directions regarding the use of life-sustaining procedures, it is my intention that this declaration be honored by my family and attending physician as the final expression of my legal right to refuse medical or surgical treatment and accept the consequences from such refusal.

I understand the full import of this declaration and I have emotional and mental capacity to make this declaration.

Signed: _____

Signed Name

_____

Printed Name

_____

City and County

_____

State

The declarant is personally known to me and I believe him (her) to be of sound mind.

_____

Witness

_____

Witness

Source: Arizona General Assembly, 1985, p. 3.

Some states have enacted living will legislation that institutionalizes the document and relieves the caregiver of the conflict of values between professional ethics and the request of the patient. The will of the patient should prevail.

It is advisable for any organization providing chronic care to constitute an ethics committee to establish organizational guidelines, increase sensitivity to the organization's responsibilities in this arena, and hear situations that do not clearly fit into the guidelines.

Research. Informed consent also becomes an important issue in the process of obtaining volunteers for research, and much research is needed in chronic care. Obtaining consent may be difficult unless the proposal is appropriately presented to the possible volunteer. Several principles have been promulgated to provide an ethical basis for research using human subjects. "The first principle is respect for persons—that is, persons capable of deciding for themselves should do so and those who are incapable of deciding should be entitled to protection. The second principle is beneficence, which requires that the investigation should minimize risk and maximize benefits. The third is justice, meaning, among other things, that the benefits as well as the burdens of research should be shared equally among potential participants. The last principle is of particular importance for patients in nursing homes, since they may be selected as potential subjects for research because of their easy availability" (Warren and others, 1986, p. 1126).

Research involving an incompetent resident of a nursing home should never be conducted without the informed consent of the subject's guardian and should be related to a topic unique to such nursing home residents. Nursing home patients should not become research subjects of convenience because of their availability.

Education of Staff and Family

In many ways the staff and family members who provide chronic care are the most intensive monitors of the quality of the care. Those being served develop trust relationships with those who provide services, and caregivers are frequently consulted before personal decisions are made. Caregivers become attuned to the responses of their clients and can detect early on the changes that might give cause for alarm. It is the responsibility of caregivers to report evidence of physical abuse, unusual anxiety, depression, or a change in response or attitude.

Caregivers need to be educated about the importance of their observations and about the correct organizational procedure that should be used to communicate an observation that might be useful (either for care planning or the monitoring of the value of services).

It has been noted that an individual who has a knowledgeable advocate has an enhanced opportunity to receive the appropriate service in timely fashion. The presence of family members as advocates serves as a constant reminder of the need for quality service.

Issues related to ethics, personal values, freedom, and paternalism are part of the complex of chronic care, irrespective of the site where services are delivered. That may be at home, in a nursing home, in an adult day health center, at a nutrition site, or on a bus from home to a service. The providers of services need to be guided by the ethical standards of the organization, as reinforced by continuing education and the modeling of ethical behavior by the organization's leadership. Chronically ill older persons can be unwittingly exposed to the indignities of paternalism, abuse, or other unethical behavior because of the desire to respond to the needs of those who are severely dependent. Maintenance of the dignity of the person requires careful attention to and review of the patterns of care to make certain they reflect the ethical standards expected of providers of chronic care.

Chapter 14

CONCLUSION:
FOUNDATIONS FOR
THE SUCCESS OF
COORDINATED CARE SYSTEMS

WHETHER OR NOT WE ARE CONSCIOUS of it, we must perform selfishly. The ways in which we treat old people today, the services and programs we pioneer, the standards we set, will determine the ways in which society perceives and treats us in our later years. If we want dignity, privacy, respect, amenities, we must provide them for others now. We must assure old people a future. The quotation, "The true test of a society (or a civilization) is in the way it treats old people" has been attributed to many—it is nevertheless true [Shore, 1987, p. 42].

The coordinated system of chronic care *can* be achieved. The knowledge and resources are available. Several groups have already demonstrated how it can be done.

For example, San Francisco's On Lok developed a system and financing pattern that is now being demonstrated at several other sites throughout the country. On Lok has shown how to utilize Medicare and Medicaid in a coordinated care system and been able to interest the Robert Wood Johnson Foundation in providing support for institution of this model at a number of locations.

St. Vincent's Hospital and Medical Center of New York demonstrated its own coordinated chronic care model and stimulated state support for its interventions to improve health care for the elderly.

Sinai Samaritan Medical Center in Milwaukee established a geriatrics institute as a center where direct services to the elderly and their families, education about aging, and research are carried on.

The Pima County model was initiated by the local Area Agency on Aging (Pima Council on Aging), which was successful in having a demonstration project continued through the resources of county government.

Mt. Zion Hospital in San Francisco integrated public and private funds to develop its model.

Brandeis University's Health Policy Center stimulated the development of the social HMO and the Life Care at Home Project and has interested major foundations in supporting innovative model programs.

It can be done.

This book has been written to stimulate interest in the development of coordinated chronic care programs, to define the characteristics of such programs, and to present examples of successful programs that are already operating.

Several additional thoughts that can contribute to the implementation of additional coordinated chronic care programs come to mind.

- The conceptual and financial issues that separate acute and chronic care must be abandoned and replaced by a health care system that responds to human caring needs in a continuum. The artificial separations reinforced by our educational institutions, delivery systems, and financing mechanisms must be dismantled. Chronic care has emerged as a central issue in health care and must incorporate curing wherever possible—and caring consistently throughout the provision of services.
- Our health care financing resources, both public and private,

need to provide for the health care needs of our people without differentiating between acute and chronic care. Eligibility for services should not be related to the potential for cure or predictions of restoration of function, but must be correlated with the need of the individual and the family.

- Public laws can and do change, and public officials are responsive to presentations that are both compassionate and factual. The demographics of our aging society have alerted lawmakers to the need for change and improvement in the delivery of care to older persons. Changes in the number of people in need will cause changes in the delivery and the financing of services. While many models of innovative programs have been demonstrated, the need for both replication of successful models and the creation of new models continues to exist.

- Incentives must be offered to make it possible for individuals to be maintained at home when that is their wish and it is compatible with the provision of services.

- Incentives for acknowledging and maintaining the very significant quality and quantity of caring provided by family members are urgently needed.

- It should be fully expected that the rapid growth of the very-old segment of our population will result in increasing demands for health services, which in turn will result in increasing the share of the gross national product that must be allocated to pay the costs of health care for the elderly. This invites unrealistic comparisons with both the costs of caring for the older cohorts in earlier years and with the costs of providing health care to younger cohorts.

- Clearly there is a need for funding from both private and public sources for research that will shed new light on the chronic health problems encountered by older people, on the best way to deliver services, and on the financing of services.

Appendix A

ORGANIZATIONS CONCERNED WITH AGING AND CHRONIC CARE

Area Agencies on Aging

National Association of Area Agencies on Aging
600 Maryland Ave. SW
West Wing, Suite 208
Washington, DC 20024
Telephone (202) 484-7520

Associations of Elderly or Disabled Persons

American Association of Retired Persons
1909 K St. NW
Washington, DC 20049
Telephone (202) 872-4700
Organization of 20 million individuals and 3,500 groups representing the interests of persons aged 50 and older, retired or otherwise. Devoted to improving every aspect of living for older people. Provides group health insurance and discounts

on services and sponsors community programs on such topics as crime prevention, defensive driving, and tax aid. Sponsors the AARP Andrus Foundation, devoted to research in gerontology. Offers special services to retired teachers through a separate National Retired Teachers Association. Maintains an online data base on aging and publishes several periodicals.

American Coalition of Citizens with Disabilities
1012 14th St. NW, Suite 901
Washington, DC 20005
Telephone (202) 628-3470
     Organization of people with physical, mental, or emotional impairment and organizations that represent them. Seeks to help disabled persons and protect their rights to education, housing, employment, transportation, and health care. Issues a number of periodic publications.

National Council of Senior Citizens
925 15th St. NW
Washington, DC 20005
Telephone (202) 347-8800
     Organization of autonomous senior citizen clubs, associations, councils, and other groups; has a combined membership of 4.5 million persons. Education and action group that supports Medicare, improved Social Security, and many other programs to aid senior citizens. Sponsors rallies, workshops, and leadership training institutes. Encourages participation in social and political-action activities. Maintains library and National Senior Citizens Education and Research Center. Publishes monthly journal.

Gerontology and Geriatrics

American Geriatrics Society
Ten Columbus Circle, Suite 1470
New York, NY 10019
Telephone (212) 582-1333
     Professional society of physicians interested in problems of the elderly. Established to encourage and promote the study

of geriatrics and medical research in the field of aging. Publishes a monthly journal and a monthly newsletter.

American Society on Aging
(Formerly Western Gerontological Society)
833 Market St., Suite 516
San Francisco, CA 94103
Telephone (415) 543-2617
Organization of health care and social service professionals, educators, researchers, students, and senior citizens that works to improve the well-being of older people through its National Training Center on Aging and other educational programs. Monitors legislation affecting the aging and issues policy recommendations to governing bodies. Maintains computer lists of members and conference attendees. Publishes *ASA Connection* bimonthly and *Generations* quarterly.

Gerontological Society of America
1411 K St. NW, Suite 300
Washington, DC 20005
Telephone (202) 393-1411
Organization of many types of professionals concerned about the well-being of older persons that promotes scientific study of the aging process, publishes information about aging, and brings together groups interested in older people. Publishes a monthly newsletter and two monthly journals.

National Council on Aging
600 Maryland Ave. SW
West Wing 100
Washington, DC 20024
Telephone (202) 479-1200
National information and consulting center that sponsors research and demonstration projects, maintains a library, and publishes widely on subjects related to aging.
Affiliated subdivisions, which have the same address, include:

National Center on Rural Aging. Established to develop social and public policies related to the needs and interests of rural older adults as well as to improve services to them. Disseminates information and promotes research and demonstration projects. Conducts training and provides technical assistance.

National Institute on Adult Day Care. Involved in planning and providing day care for older persons through training and technical assistance to providers. Lobbies for approved public policy decisions; surveys state day care standards, regulations, and legislation.

National Institute on Community-Based Long-Term Care. Advocate for promotion and development of community-based chronic care systems and public policies supporting them. Maintains speakers' bureau, offers educational sessions, publishes quarterly newsletter.

National Institute of Senior Centers. Assists senior centers, organizations, and communities in developing new centers and upgrading existing ones. Promotes professionalism in the senior center field, advocates for national standards, provides training and publications.

National Institute of Senior Housing. Seeks to organize and maintain a national response to the need for affordable, decent housing and living arrangements for older adults. Conducts workshops, symposiums, and training and serves as a clearinghouse on housing options for the elderly.

National Voluntary Organizations for Independent Living for the Aging. Encourages cooperation between voluntary organizations and the public to improve the lives of older people through in-home and community-based health and social services. Sponsors workshops, seminars, and projects.

Home Care

American Association for Continuity of Care
1101 Connecticut Ave. SW, Suite 700
Washington, DC 20036
Telephone (202) 857-1194

Health care professionals involved in discharge planning, social work, hospital administration, home care, chronic care, home health agencies, and continuity of care. Studies and researches health care issues, including those related to Medicare. Publishes bimonthly newsletter and annual directory.

American Federation of Home Health Agencies
1320 Fenwick Ln., Suite 500
Silver Spring, MD 20910
Telephone (301) 588-1454
Association of agencies providing therapeutic services such as nursing and speech or physical therapy in the home, having as its purpose promotion of health by influencing public policy. Lobbies with Congress and the Health Care Financing Administration and helps members work with their fiscal intermediaries. Conducts seminars and publishes bimonthly gazette.

Home Health Services and Staffing Association
815 Connecticut Ave. NW, Suite 206
Washington, DC 20006
Telephone (202) 331-4437
Association of proprietary home care organizations that provide health care services in patients' homes and supplemental nursing services in institutions. Acts as a representative regarding federal and state legislation affecting home care and supplemental nursing services and works to develop a national health policy.

National Association for Home Care
519 C St. NE
Washington, DC 20002
Telephone (202) 547-7424
Seeks to develop and promote high standards of patient care in home care services, including home health aides. Seeks to affect legislative policies and regulatory processes, to increase visibility of home care services, and to gather and disseminate home care data. Offers legal and accounting consultation services, conducts market research, and compiles statistics. Sponsors educational programs and issues several publications.

National Homecaring Council
235 Park Ave. S
New York, NY 10003
Telephone (212) 674-4990

Promotes understanding of the values of homemaker and home health services, conducts a consumer education and protection program, provides a central source of information, encourages establishment and expansion of community home health services, promotes development of standards, and administers an agency approval/accreditation program. Maintains a library and issues several periodic publications.

Hospice

National Hospice Organization
1901 N. Fort Meyer Dr., Suite 902
Arlington, VA 22209
Telephone (703) 243-5900

Promotes standards of care in program planning and implementation for hospices, collects data for the purpose of demonstrating national trends in the hospice movement, encourages recognized medical and other health-education institutions to provide instruction in hospice care of the terminally ill and members of their families. Conducts educational and training programs. Maintains a library and issues several periodic publications.

Hospital Administration

American Hospital Association
840 Lake Shore Dr.
Chicago, IL 60611
Telephone (312) 280-6000

Carries out research and education projects in such areas as health administration, hospital economics, hospital facilities and design, and community relations. Represents hospitals in national legislation. Offers programs for institutional effectiveness review and technology assessment. Maintains health care administration library and issues a number of periodicals.

Specialty subdivisions of the AHA, which have the same address, include:

American College of Healthcare Executives. Professional society for hospital and health service administrators. Maintains data base of personal and career data for its members. Holds seminars on health care management. Maintains numerous committees and task forces, conducts research programs, and compiles statistics. Issues several periodic publications.

Division of Ambulatory Care. Serves hospitals and other health care providers with interests in ambulatory care, emergency care, home care, HMOs, and hospices. Represents views of its institutional members to Congress and regulatory agencies. Conducts conferences, seminars, and research. Publishes bimonthly journal.

Special Constituency Section of Aging and Long Term Care. Promotes recognition, growth, and support for institutions having chronic care units or community-based chronic care and special services for the aging.

Catholic Health Association of the United States
4455 Woodson Rd.
St. Louis, MO 63134
Telephone (314) 427-2500
Established to provide leadership to Catholic health organizations through analysis of trends and developments in the health field, contribute to development and implementation of optimal programs by Catholic health organizations, and represent Catholic health services to public and private agencies. Maintains library on health care administration and issues several periodic publications.

Law and Aging

National Senior Citizens Law Center
2025 M St. NW, Suite 400
Washington, DC 20036
Telephone (202) 887-5280

Legal services support center specializing in the legal problems of the elderly. Acts as an advocate on behalf of elderly poor clients in litigation and administrative affairs. Sponsors conferences and workshops on areas of the law affecting the elderly. Maintains library and issues various publications.

Mental Health and Mental Retardation

Accreditation Council for Development
of Services for Mentally Retarded and
Other Developmentally Disabled Persons
4435 Wisconsin Ave. NW, Suite 202
Washington, DC 20016
Telephone (202) 363-2811

Nonprofit organization devoted to the improvement of services to the mentally retarded and otherwise developmentally disabled. Assesses agency compliance with standards (on request). Offers accreditation to agencies and workshops on improving standards. Publishes newsletter and *Standards for Services for Developmentally Disabled Individuals.*

Association for Retarded Citizens
P.O. Box 6109
Arlington, TX 76006
Telephone (817) 640-0204

Organization of parents, professional workers, and others interested in persons who are mentally retarded that works at local, state, and national levels to promote services, research public understanding, and further legislation on their behalf. Maintains library and issues periodic publications.

Mental Retardation Association of America
211 E. 300 South St., Suite 212
Salt Lake City, UT 84111
Telephone (801) 328-1575

Independent volunteer organization of associations of persons working in the field of mental retardation. Works for legislation on behalf of the retarded, public understanding, and the development of small-group homes.

National Alliance for the Mentally Ill
1901 N. Fort Meyer Dr., Suite 500
Arlington, VA 22209
Telephone (703) 524-7600
    Alliance of self-help/advocacy groups concerned with the welfare of the severely and chronically mentally ill. Works to provide families and the public with sound information about mental illness. Monitors quality of treatment. Promotes research in the neurosciences and rehabilitation. Issues periodic publications.

National Mental Health Association
1021 Prince St.
Arlington, VA 22314
Telephone (703) 684-7722
    Consumer advocacy group devoted to advancement of mental health and promotion of research to discover new and better ways to treat and prevent mental illness.

Nursing

American Nurses' Association
2420 Pershing Rd.
Kansas City, MO 64108
Telephone (816) 474-5720
    National association for registered nurses, representing nearly 200,000 individuals, 53 state groups, and 860 local groups. Sponsors subdivisions dealing with research, political action, economics and general welfare, human rights, education, and many nursing specialties, including gerontology. Sponsors annual awards for outstanding contributions to nursing. Issues a number of regular periodicals.

National Federation of Licensed Practical Nurses
P.O. Box 11038
214 Driver St.
Durham, NC 27703
Telephone (919) 596-9609
    Federation of state associations of licensed practical and

vocational nurses established to serve and foster the ideal of comprehensive nursing care for the ill and aged, to improve standards of practice, and to secure recognition and effective utilization of LPNs. Acts as a clearinghouse for information on practical nursing and cooperates with other groups concerned with better patient care. Maintains a data bank and a loan program. Publishes quarterly journal.

National League for Nursing
Ten Columbus Circle
New York, NY 10019
Telephone (212) 582-1022
    Works to assess nursing needs, improve organized nursing services and nursing education, and foster collaboration between nursing and other health and community services. Provides tests used for selection of applicants to schools of nursing, evaluation of student progress, and nursing service. Accredits nursing education programs and community nursing services. Maintains and distributes data on nursing profession. Conducts studies and demonstration projects on community planning for nursing, nursing service, and nursing education.

Visiting Nurse Associations of America
518 17th St., #388
Denver, CO 80202
Telephone (303) 629-8622
    Affiliation of branches of the Visiting Nurse Association and Visiting Nurse Services established to develop competitive strength among health care agencies, particularly those supported by hospitals and corporations. Develops business resources and economic programs through marketing and contracting. Issues radio and television public service announcements and offers workshops and training programs.

Nursing Homes

American Association of Homes for the Aging
1129 20th St. NW, Suite 400
Washington, DC 20036
Telephone (202) 296-5960

Affiliation of voluntary nonprofit and government housing and health-related services for the elderly. Organized to protect the interests of residents of specialized housing for the elderly. Believes that chronic care should be geared to individual needs and should offer a broad spectrum of service levels, ranging from independent living at home to full-time nursing care. Provides liaison with Congress and federal agencies, educational programs, a group purchasing program, and insurance programs. Issues several periodic publications.

American College of Health Care Administrators
8120 Woodmont Ave., Suite 200
Bethesda, MD 20814
Telephone (301) 652-8384

Organization of persons actively engaged in administration of chronic care institutions, medical administration, or activities designed to improve the quality of nursing home administration. Certifies members' ability to meet and maintain a standard of competence in administration and works to develop nursing home standards and a code of ethics and standards of education and training. Encourages research in all aspects of geriatrics. Maintains a library and sponsors education programs and regional seminars. Maintains placement service. Publishes several periodicals.

American Health Care Association
1200 15th St. NW
Washington, DC 20005
Telephone (202) 833-2050

Federation of state associations of chronic care facilities. Promotes professional standards; focuses on issues of availability, quality, and affordability. Conducts seminars and continuing education for nursing home personnel. Maintains liaison with government agencies, Congress, and professional associations. Presents awards and compiles statistics. Publishes several periodicals.

American Medical Directors Association
1200 15th St. NW
Washington, DC 20005
Telephone (202) 659-3148

Organization of physicians and allied personnel providing care in chronic care facilities. Sponsors continuing medical education in geriatrics. Promotes improved geriatric care. Publishes newsletter three times a year.

National Foundation for Long Term Health Care
1200 15th St. NW
Washington, DC 20005
Telephone (202) 833-2050

Funds research into issues of chronic health care and the elderly and presents up-to-date research findings through periodic issue papers focusing on geriatric care. Seeks to improve the public perception of chronic care through educational and media programs. Conducts symposiums for professionals. Maintains library and compiles statistics. Publishes training materials and periodicals.

Nutrition

American Dietetic Association
430 Michigan Ave.
Chicago, IL 60611
Telephone (312) 280-5000

Professional organization of dietitians in hospitals and other institutions that seeks to provide direction and leadership for dietetic practice, education, and research. Sets and approves standards of education and experience through internships and coordinated undergraduate, M.S. and Ph.D. programs. Provides career guidance and scholarships and awards through the ADA Foundation. Publishes monthly journal.

American Society for Parenteral and Enteral Nutrition
8605 Cameron St., Suite 500
Silver Spring, MD 20910
Telephone (301) 587-6315

Dedicated to fostering good nutritional support of patients during hospitalization and rehabilitation. Educates health care professionals at all levels and encourages the development of improved patient care. Compiles statistics and publishes journals and educational materials.

National Association of Meal Programs
204 E St. NE
Washington, DC 20002
Telephone (202) 547-6340
  Association of agencies involved in delivery of nutritionally balanced meals to disabled and homebound elderly persons. Advocates community-based, home-delivered, and congregate meal programs, provides technical assistance in establishing new programs, develops organizational materials, conducts training seminars. Publishes newsletter and technical bulletins.

National Association of Nutrition and Aging
P.O. Box 505
Frankfort, IN 46401
Telephone (317) 659-1907
  Organization of directors and staff of home-delivered and congregate meal programs established to raise the standards of the profession among members, encourage communication between aging services programs, federal agencies, and governmental bodies, and promote development of programs to support aging services programs. Has developed national standards for home-delivered and congregate meal programs. Issues several publications.

Social Work

National Association of Social Workers
7981 Eastern Ave.
Silver Spring, MD 20910
Telephone (301) 565-0333
  Association of professional social workers formed to create standards of practice and advocate sound public policies through political and social action. Provides membership services that include continuing education opportunities and extensive professional publications. Maintains a library and computerized information data base. Persons enrolled in accredited social work study programs are eligible for student memberships.

Society for Hospital Social Work Directors
American Hospital Association Building
840 Lake Shore Dr.
Chicago, IL 60611
Telephone (312) 280-6414

Organization of directors of social work departments in hospitals having as its purpose the improvement and extension of adequate health services for all persons and the development of effective social work administration in health care facilities through educational programs and exchange of ideas. Publishes *Social Work Administration* bimonthly and *Discharge Planning Update* quarterly.

Special Focus Organizations

Alzheimer's Disease and Related
Disorders Association (ADRDA)
70 E. Lake St., Suite 600
Chicago, IL 60601
Telephone (312) 853-3060

Organization to promote research to find the cause, treatment, and cure for the disease and to provide educational programs for the public, the media, and health care professionals. Represents continuing care needs of the affected population before government and social service agencies. Publishes a newsletter and a quarterly.

American Protestant Health Association
1701 E. Woodfield Rd.
Schaumberg, IL 60195
Telephone (312) 843-2701

Organization of Protestant health and welfare institutional chaplains that maintains a computerized data base and mailing list and issues periodic information in cassette and published formats.

Church of the Brethren Homes and Hospital
1451 Dundee Ave.
Elgin, IL 60120
Telephone (312) 742-5100

Association of administrators and board members of the Brethren Homes for the Aged (twenty-four) and one hospital, organized to share their common concerns and programs of service to hospitalized or aging people.

National Caucus and Center on Black Aged
1424 K St. NW, Suite 500
Washington, DC 20005
Telephone (202) 637-8400
Seeks to enhance the quality of life for aging Americans, particularly blacks. Advocates changes in federal and state laws to improve the economic, health, and social status of low-income senior citizens. Sponsors an employment program. Owns and operates rental housing for the elderly and conducts training programs in gerontology and housing management.

National Hispanic Council on Aging
2713 Ontario Rd. NW
Washington, DC 20024
Telephone (202) 265-1288
Organization of individuals who work in administration, planning, direct services, research, and education on behalf of the aging. Fosters the well-being of the Hispanic elderly through activities in all these areas. Compiles research data on the Hispanic elderly. Provides a network of persons and agencies concerned for Hispanic elderly and testifies at hearings. Publishes a quarterly newsletter.

National Indian Council on Aging
P.O. Box 2088
Albuquerque, NM 87103
Telephone (505) 242-9505
Established to bring about improved, comprehensive services to Indian and Alaskan native elderly and to act as a focal point for articulation of the needs of these groups. Disseminates information on Indian aging programs, provides technical assistance and training opportunities to tribal organizations, and conducts research on the needs of the Indian elderly. Publishes a monthly journal and various proceedings, reports, and monographs.

National Pacific/Asian Resource Center on Aging
Colorado Building
1341 G St. NW, Suite 311
Washington, DC 20005
Telephone (202) 393-7838

Established to ensure and improve the delivery of health and social services to elderly Pacific/Asians, to increase the capabilities of community-based services, and to include Pacific/Asians in planning and organizational activities. Provides technical assistance, compiles statistics, maintains library, and issues several periodic publications.

North American Association of
Jewish Homes and Housing for the Aged
2525 Centerville Rd.
Dallas, TX 75228
Telephone (214) 327-4503

Organization representing nonprofit charitable Jewish homes, retirement homes and nursing homes, independent living or shared quarters, geriatric hospitals, and special facilities for Jewish aged and chronically ill. Conducts institutes and conferences, undertakes legislative activities, and compiles statistics. Publishes a quarterly report and biennial directory.

Almost all of these organizations hold an annual conference for members, either independently or in conjunction with some other professional group.

Appendix B

SUMMARY OF MEDICARE, MEDICAID, AND PRIVATE INSURANCE COVERAGE FOR CHRONIC CARE

CONTRARY TO THE EXPECTATIONS of the public, and especially of older persons, Medicare is essentially an acute care program and provides only nominal resources for chronic care. The major part of the public responsibility for funding chronic care is through the Medicaid program, and because Medicaid eligibility is restricted to persons having low incomes, achieving such eligibility often requires the reduction of assets known as "spending down." In other words, an individual or family is forced to become impoverished in order to benefit from the program. At this time few older persons carry private insurance to protect them against the heavy financial burdens of chronic care. Consequently, extended long-term care or disability that requires personal and nursing care often results in financial ruin for the elderly. This problem will become more acute as persons 65 and older become a larger proportion of the population.

Brief descriptions of Medicare and Medicaid coverage and of the two major types of relevant private insurance, prepared by the U.S. Senate Special Committee on Aging (1987), will clarify the limitations of these payment programs.

227

Medicare

The Medicare program, which insures almost 98% of all older Americans without regard to income or assets, does not cover either long-term or custodial care. Primarily it provides acute care for those age 65 and older, particularly hospital and surgical care and accompanying periods of recovery. Further, in order to receive reimbursement under Medicare, the patient must be in need of skilled nursing care (SNF) on a daily basis for treatment related to a condition for which he or she was hospitalized. The SNF benefit is subject to a daily patient co-payment after the 20th day of care. In 1986, the co-payment was $61.50 per day, rising to $65 in 1987. The program pays for neither intermediate care nor custodial care in a nursing home.

Even though Medicare coverage of home health care is only for shorter periods of care and only for treatment of an acute care condition or for post-acute care, the Medicare home health benefit is the fastest growing component of the Medicare program.

Home health services covered under Medicare include the following:

- Part time or intermittent nursing care provided by, or under the supervision of, a registered professional nurse
- Physical, occupational, or speech therapy
- Medical social services provided under the direction of a physician
- Medical supplies and equipment (other than drugs and medicines)
- Medical services provided by an intern or resident enrolled in a teaching program in a hospital affiliated or under contract with a home health agency

- Part time or intermittent services provided by a home health aide, as permitted by regulations

To qualify for home health services, the Medicare beneficiary must be confined to the home and under the care of a physician. In addition, the person must be in need of part time or intermittent skilled nursing care or physical or speech therapy. Services must be provided by a home health agency certified to participate under Medicare, according to a plan of treatment prescribed and reviewed by a physician. The patient is not subject to any cost sharing, e.g., deductibles or co-insurance for covered home care.

In addition to these SNF and home health care benefits, Medicare covers a range of long-term care services, and especially home care services, for terminally ill beneficiaries. These services, authorized in 1982 and referred to as Medicare's hospice benefits, are available to beneficiaries with a life expectancy of six months or less. Hospice care benefits include nursing care, therapy services, medical social services, home health aide services, physician services, counseling, and short-term inpatient care [pp. 270–271].

Medicaid

The Medicaid program, which provides medical assistance for certain low income persons, excludes most older Americans. Medicaid has nonetheless become the primary source of public funds for nursing home care. Approximately 80% of all public expenditures for nursing home care is paid by Medicaid and 48% of all nursing home residents are Medicaid beneficiaries. Each state administers its own program and, subject to federal guidelines, determines the Medicaid income eligibility standard.

State Medicaid programs are required by federal law to cover the categorically needy, that is, all persons receiving assistance under the Aid to Families with Dependent Children (AFDC) Program and most people receiving assistance under the Supplemental Security Income (SSI) Program. States may also cover persons who would be eligible for cash assistance, except when they are residents in medical institutions, such as skilled nursing facilities (SNFs) or intermediate care facilities (ICFs).

In addition, states may, at their discretion, cover the medically needy, that is, persons whose income and resources are large enough to cover daily living expenses, according to income levels set by the state, but are not large enough to pay for medical care. These state variations mean persons with identical circumstances may be eligible to receive Medicaid benefits in one state, but not in another.

To control costs and to provide a range of community-based services to the Medicaid-eligible population, many states have applied to the Department of Health and Human Services (DHHS) for section 2176 Medicaid waivers. In 1981, Congress established these waivers, giving DHHS the authority to waive certain Medicaid requirements to allow the states to broaden coverage to include a range of community-based services for persons who, without such services, would require a level of care provided in an SNF or ICF. Services covered under the 2176 waiver include case management, homemaker, home health aide, personal care, adult day care, rehabilitation, respite, and others [pp. 268–269].

Private Insurance

1. Medigap. Seventy-two percent of older Americans purchase supplemental medical insurance, or medigap policies. About half of this supplemental coverage is provided on a group basis—mainly through retirees' former employers—and about half is purchased individually. These policies are typically designed to supplement Medicare's coverage of acute care costs, not long-term care costs.

To illustrate, some medigap policies cover the daily co-payment from the 20th to the 100th day of an approved stay in a Medicare SNF. Others provide coverage for skilled care, as defined by Medicare, in a certified facility for stays of 100 to 365 days, or longer. The value of the medigap coverage for long-term care, however, is very limited. These policies generally cover a very small fraction of total nursing home costs and an even smaller portion of home health or custodial care costs.

2. Long-Term Care Insurance Policies. Currently, only about 1% of the nation's long-term care expenditures is paid for by private insurance. A 1986 survey by the Health Insurance Association of America found that 12 companies offered individual indemnity life insurance and that there were 130,000 policyholders with an average age of 75. These policies typically offer indemnity benefits for three years of care in a licensed nursing care facility. Ten of the 12 policies continue coverage after the need for skilled nursing care is fulfilled and the long-term care needs become custodial in nature [p. 274].

Appendix C

ARIZONA MINIMUM
ASSESSMENT INSTRUMENT

ARIZONA DEPARTMENT OF ECONOMIC SECURITY

Aging and Adult Administration, 950A

ARIZONA MINIMUM ASSESSMENT

I. IDENTIFYING INFORMATION

A. *(If Assessment Time, write the actual Assessment Time in box)*

Assessment Time *(In minutes)*

☐ New Application ☐ Eligibility Redetermination

B. SOCIAL SECURITY NUMBER

C. DATE *(MM-DD-YY)*

D. CLIENT NAME *(Last, First, MI)*

E. BIRTHDATE *(MM-DD-YY)*

AGE

F. SEX
☐ Male ☐ Female

G. COUNTY

H. PHONE NO.

I. ADDRESS *(No., Street, Apt. or Space No., City, ZIP)*

J. SOURCE OF REFERRAL

☐ 1. Client
☐ 2. Family
☐ 3. Friend
☐ 4. Hospital
☐ 5. Agency
☐ 6. Other _____
☐ 7. Confidential APS

K. MARITAL STATUS

☐ 1. Married
☐ 2. Separated
☐ 3. Single
☐ 4. Divorced
☐ 5. Widowed

L. EDUCATION LEVEL

☐ 1. 8th Grade or Less
☐ 2. Some High School
☐ 3. High School Graduate
☐ 4. Some Post Secondary
☐ 5. College Graduate

M. ETHNICITY

☐ 1. Caucasian *(Non-Hisp.)*
☐ 2. Hispanic
☐ 3. Black *(Non-Hisp.)*
☐ 4. Asian *(Non-Hisp.)*
☐ 5. Amer. Ind. *(Non-Hisp.)*
☐ 6. Other _____
☐ 7. Unknown

N. PRIMARY SPOKEN LANGUAGE

☐ 1. English
☐ 2. Spanish *(Can Speak English)*
☐ 3. Spanish *(Can't Speak English)*
☐ 4. Native Amer. *(Can Speak English)*
☐ 5. Native Amer. *(Can't Speak English)*
☐ 6. Other *(Can Speak English)*
☐ 7. Other *(Can't Speak English)*

O. PERSONAL/LEGAL STATUS

☐ 1. Independent *(Self Responsible)*
☐ 2. Dependent Child *(Under 18 Years)*
☐ 3. Court-appointed Guardian
☐ 4. Court-appointed Conservator
☐ 5. Power-of-attorney *(Rep. Payee)*

P. LIVING ARRANGEMENT

☐ Rent ☐ Own _____

☐ 1. Private Home/Apartment
☐ 2. Mobil Home
☐ 3. Room
☐ 4. Board and Care Home *(Unlicensed)*
☐ 5. Foster Care Home
☐ 6. Supervisory Care
☐ 7. Nursing Home
☐ 8. Other

Q. HOUSEHOLD COMPOSITION

Number in Household ___
Number in Family ___

Client lives
☐ 1. Alone
☐ 2. With Spouse or Equivalent Only
☐ 3. With Family
☐ 4. With Others

R. ELIGIBILITY

☐ Medicare
☐ Title XX-ELD
☐ Title XX-HC
☐ Title XX
☐ Title XX-DD
☐ Title III
☐ SPP Dir. Pay
☐ SPP-HMKR
☐ SPP-HH
☐ SPP-VNS

☐ AHCCCS
☐ Veterans
☐ 3rd Party Pay
☐ H/Health Mdc.
☐ County Only
☐ SSI
☐ Other

S. SUBSIDIZED HOUSING

☐ Yes
☐ No

	STATUS	REASON	PROVIDER CODE	EFFECTIVE DATE	REVIEW DATE	AUTHORIZED UNIT(S)	MAXIMUM PER MONTH
Direct Pay Housekeeper							$
Housekeeper							$
Home Health Aid							$
Visiting Nurse							$

SOURCE OF INCOME	NAME OF PERSON RECEIVING	GROSS AMOUNT	FREQUENCY	NET AMOUNT
		$		$
		$		$
MONTHLY TOTAL		$		$

APPLICANT/CLIENT CERTIFICATION. I certify by my signature or mark that I understand my rights and responsibilities, and that the information provided on this form, as it relates to my request and eligibility, is true and correct according to my knowledge and belief.

APPLICANT/CLIENT SIGNATURE _____ DATE _____

AGENCY NAME							PHONE NO.

II. INSTRUMENTAL ACTIVITIES OF DAILY LIFE (IADL)

Circle the appropriate number for Status, Source of Help and Client Needs. Circle N or Y if client uses Assistive Devices or has a Problem

STATUS
1 = Independent
2 = Assistance
3 = Dependent

USES ASSISTIVE DEVICES Y = Yes N = No

SOURCE OF HELP
1 = None
2 = Spouse
3 = Parent
4 = Daughter
5 = Son
6 = Sibling
7 = Other Relative
8 = Friend/Neighbor
9 = Paid Help
10 = Volunteer
11 = Agency

PROBLEM Y = Yes N = No

CLIENT NEEDS
1 = Human Assistance
2 = Assistive Devices
3 = Education/Training
4 = Evaluation
5 = Other

	STATUS	USES ASSISTIVE DEVICES	SOURCE OF HELP	PROBLEM	CLIENT NEEDS
A. Medication Use	1 2 3	N Y	1 2 3 4 5 6 7 8 9 10 11	N Y	1 2 3 4 5
B. Meal Preparation	1 2 3	N Y	1 2 3 4 5 6 7 8 9 10 11	N Y	1 2 3 4 5
C. Shopping	1 2 3	N Y	1 2 3 4 5 6 7 8 9 10 11	N Y	1 2 3 4 5
D. Financial Management	1 2 3	N Y	1 2 3 4 5 6 7 8 9 10 11	N Y	1 2 3 4 5
E. Telephone Use ☐ No Telephone	1 2 3	N Y	1 2 3 4 5 6 7 8 9 10 11	N Y	1 2 3 4 5
F. Transportation	1 2 3	N Y	1 2 3 4 5 6 7 8 9 10 11	N Y	1 2 3 4 5
G. Housework	1 2 3	N Y	1 2 3 4 5 6 7 8 9 10 11	N Y	1 2 3 4 5
H. Laundry	1 2 3	N Y	1 2 3 4 5 6 7 8 9 10 11	N Y	1 2 3 4 5

IADL COMMENTS

A. Medication Use

B. Meal Preparation
(Planning and preparing)

C. Shopping *(Carrying bags, putting in cupboards, etc.)*

D. Financial Management *(Competency to budget, banking, paying bills, etc.)*

E. Telephone Use *(Picking up phone, dialing, obtaining numbers, replacing phone)*

F. Transportation *(To and from places, enter and exit vehicles)*

G. Housework *(Dusting, mopping, vacuuming, cleaning bathroom, etc.)*

H. Laundry *(Sorting, changing, storing, transferring, etc.)*

III. PERSONAL ACTIVITIES OF DAILY LIVING (PADL)

Circle the appropriate number for Status, Source of Help and Client Needs. Circle N or Y if client uses Assistive Devices or has a Problem

STATUS
1 = Independent
2 = Assistance
3 = Dependent

USES ASSISTIVE DEVICES — Y = Yes, N = No

SOURCE OF HELP
1 = None
2 = Spouse
3 = Parent
4 = Daughter
5 = Son
6 = Sibling
7 = Other Relative
8 = Friend/Neighbor
9 = Paid Help
10 = Volunteer
11 = Agency

PROBLEM — Y = Yes, N = No

CLIENT NEEDS
1 = Human Assistance
2 = Assistive Devices
3 = Education/Training
4 = Evaluation
5 = Other

	STATUS	USES ASSISTIVE DEVICES	SOURCE OF HELP	PROBLEM	CLIENT NEEDS
A. Bathing and Grooming	1 2 3	N Y	1 2 3 4 5 6 7 8 9 10 11	N Y	1 2 3 4 5
B. Dressing	1 2 3	N Y	1 2 3 4 5 6 7 8 9 10 11	N Y	1 2 3 4 5
C. Ambulation (In-home)	1 2 3	N Y	1 2 3 4 5 6 7 8 9 10 11	N Y	1 2 3 4 5
D. Ambulation (Out-of-home)	1 2 3	N Y	1 2 3 4 5 6 7 8 9 10 11	N Y	1 2 3 4 5
E. Transfer (In-home)	1 2 3	N Y	1 2 3 4 5 6 7 8 9 10 11	N Y	1 2 3 4 5
F. Transfer (Out-of-home)	1 2 3	N Y	1 2 3 4 5 6 7 8 9 10 11	N Y	1 2 3 4 5
G. Eating	1 2 3	N Y	1 2 3 4 5 6 7 8 9 10 11	N Y	1 2 3 4 5
H. Toileting (In-home)	1 2 3	N Y	1 2 3 4 5 6 7 8 9 10 11	N Y	1 2 3 4 5
I. Toileting (Out-of-home)	1 2 3	N Y	1 2 3 4 5 6 7 8 9 10 11	N Y	1 2 3 4 5

PADL COMMENTS

A. Bathing and Grooming
(Showering, bathing, hair, teeth, nails, etc.)

B. Dressing *(Obtaining clothes, putting on braces and prosthetics)*		
C. Ambulation *(In-home) (Going from place to place)*		
D. Ambulation *(Out-of-home) (Going from place to place)*		
E. Transfer *(In-home) (Chair to bed)*		
F. Transfer *(Out-of-home) (Chair to couch)*		
G. Eating *(Using fork, spoon, knife, etc.)*		
H. Toileting *(In-home) (Transferring, adjust clothing, hygiene, etc.)*		
I. Toileting *(Out-of-home) (Transferring, adjust clothing, hygiene, etc.)*		

IV. PHYSICAL IMPAIRMENT AND ILLNESS (PII)

Circle appropriate number and circle N or Y if uses Assistive Devices	1 = Continent 2 = Periodic Incontinence 3 = Complete Incontinence			USES ASSISTIVE DEVICES N = No Y = Yes	Circle appropriate number and circle N or Y if uses Assistive Device	1 = Adequate 2 = Moderate Impairment 3 = Severe Impairment			USES ASSISTIVE DEVICES N = No Y = Yes
A. Bladder	1	2	3	N Y	C. Vision	1	2	3	N Y
B. Bowel	1	2	3	N Y	D. Hearing	1	2	3	N Y

PII COMMENTS

A. Bladder

C. Vision

B. Bowel

D. Hearing

E. Medical Conditions *(Check all appropriate boxes)*

1. Hematologic Disorders
   - ☐ a. Anemia
   - ☐ b. Leukemia
   - ☐ c. Other *(Specify)*

2. Cardiovascular Disorders
   - ☐ a. Angina
   - ☐ b. Congestive Heart Failure
   - ☐ c. Heart Attack
   - ☐ d. Hypertension
   - ☐ e. Stroke
   - ☐ f. Other *(Specify)*

a. Arthritis
- [ ] a.
- [ ] b. Back Problems
- [ ] c. Broken Bone, Fracture
- [ ] d. Joint Replacement
- [ ] e. Other *(Specify)*

a. Autism
- [ ] a.
- [ ] b. Brain Damage
- [ ] c. Cerebral Palsy
- [ ] d. Convulsive Disorders
- [ ] e. Epilepsy
- [ ] f. Mental Retardation
- [ ] g. Multiple Sclerosis/Dystrophy
- [ ] h. Organic Brain Changes *(Dementia, Alzheimer)*
- [ ] i. Paralysis
- [ ] j. Parkinson's Disease
- [ ] k. Sleep Disorders
- [ ] l. Other *(Specify)*

5. Pulmonary
- [ ] a. Asthma
- [ ] b. Chronic Obstructive Disease
- [ ] c. Emphysema
- [ ] d. Other *(Specify)*

6. Urologic
- [ ] a. Bladder/Kidney Problems
- [ ] b. Male Problems
- [ ] c. Other *(Specify)*

7. Psychiatric
- [ ] a. Alcohol Abuse
- [ ] b. Drug Abuse
- [ ] c. Other *(Specify)*

8. Gastrointestinal
- [ ] a. Colitis
- [ ] b. Constipation
- [ ] c. Diarrhea
- [ ] d. GI Bleeding
- [ ] e. Hemorrhoids
- [ ] f. Stomach and Intestinal Problems
- [ ] g. Ulcers
- [ ] h. Other *(Specify)*

E. Medical Conditions (Continued)

9. Ophthalmologic
   - ☐ a. Cataract
   - ☐ b. Glaucoma
   - ☐ c. Other (Specify)

10. Gynecology
    - ☐ a. Female Problems
    - ☐ b. Other (Specify)

11. General Medical Problems
    - ☐ a. AIDS
    - ☐ b. Allergy
    - ☐ c. Bruises
    - ☐ d. Cancer
    - ☐ e. Chronic Pain
    - ☐ f. Communicable Disease
    - ☐ g. Decubitus
    - ☐ h. Eczema
    - ☐ i. Edema
    - ☐ j. Psoriasis
    - ☐ k. Tumor
    - ☐ l. Other (Specify)

12. Metabolic
    - ☐ a. Diabetes
    - ☐ b. Thyroid
    - ☐ c. Other (Specify)

F. Emergency Information

	NAME	ADDRESS	PHONE NO
Physician			
Persons to Notify	NAME	ADDRESS	PHONE NO.
	NAME	ADDRESS	PHONE NO.

☐ No ☐ Yes If yes, how many times. _____ Number of nights in hospital. _____

G. Medications

1. Number of prescribed medications taken. ☐ _(List)_ _____

_____

_____

_____

_____

2. Number of over-the-counter medications taken. ☐ _(List)_ _____

_____

_____

_____

_____

3. Special diet ☐ No ☐ Yes: If yes, describe _____

V. PROGNOSIS FOR SUPPORT

☐ Check if None

Sources of Support	Source of Help		Household Member		Rarely - 1 x/mo. = 1 Occasionally - 2 or 3 x/mo. = 2 Frequently - 4 or more/mo. = 3			Anticipated Changes in Next Six (6) Mos. 1 = decrease 2 = same 3 = increase		
	No	Yes	No	Yes	1	2	3	1	2	3
A. Spouse/Equivalent	☐	☐	☐	☐	☐	☐	☐	☐	☐	☐
B. Parent	☐	☐	☐	☐	☐	☐	☐	☐	☐	☐
C. Daughter	☐	☐	☐	☐	☐	☐	☐	☐	☐	☐
D. Son	☐	☐	☐	☐	☐	☐	☐	☐	☐	☐
E. Sibling	☐	☐	☐	☐	☐	☐	☐	☐	☐	☐
F. Other Relative	☐	☐	☐	☐	☐	☐	☐	☐	☐	☐
G. Friend/Neighbor	☐	☐	☐	☐	☐	☐	☐	☐	☐	☐
H. Privately Paid Help	☐	☐	☐	☐	☐	☐	☐	☐	☐	☐
I. Community Volunteer	☐	☐						☐	☐	☐
J. Agency	☐	☐						☐	☐	☐

Comments _____

VI. ASSISTIVE DEVICES

Check **one** box for each item. If more than one code applies, check highest number only.

	No Need 1	Has No Problem 2	Has Possible Problem 3	Needs 4
A. Eye Glasses/Contacts	☐	☐	☐	☐
B. Hearing Aid	☐	☐	☐	☐
C. Phone Amplifier	☐	☐	☐	☐
D. Dentures	☐	☐	☐	☐
E. External Prosthetic Device(s)	☐	☐	☐	☐
F. Cane/Quad Cane	☐	☐	☐	☐
G. Walker/Crutches	☐	☐	☐	☐
H. Manual/Electric Wheelchair	☐	☐	☐	☐
I. Tub/Shower Seat	☐	☐	☐	☐
J. Raised Toilet Seat	☐	☐	☐	☐
K. Commode Chair	☐	☐	☐	☐
L. Urinal Bed Pan	☐	☐	☐	☐
M. Handrails, Grab Bars	☐	☐	☐	☐
N. Transfer Equipment	☐	☐	☐	☐
O. Medication Reminder System	☐	☐	☐	☐
P. Colostomy/Ileostomy Equipment	☐	☐	☐	☐
Q. Foley Catheter Equipment	☐	☐	☐	☐
R. Oxygen Therapy Equipment	☐	☐	☐	☐
S. Hospital Bed	☐	☐	☐	☐
T. Emergency Notification Equipment	☐	☐	☐	☐
U. Other Assistive Devices	☐	☐	☐	☐

Comments ——————

VII. PSYCHOSOCIAL (PS)

A. Cognitions *(Concentration/recent memory/past memory/orientation/functioning and self care)*

☐ 1. Unimpaired
☐ 2. Minor to Moderate Impairment
☐ 3. Severe Impairment

Comments _____

B. Adequacy of Social Contacts *(As perceived by client. Is client satisfied with the amount of contact he/she has with family and friends)*

☐ 1. Adequate
☐ 2. Inadequate

Comments _____

C. Language Comprehension *(Understanding)*

☐ 1. Unimpaired
☐ 2. Minor to moderate Impairment
☐ 3. Severe Impairment

Comments _____

☐ 1. Unimpaired
☐ 2. Minor to Moderate Impairment
☐ 3. Severe Impairment

Comments _____

E. Behavior

Behavior	Sign Present		If yes, reported by			
☐ Check if None	No	Yes	Client	Assessor	Significant Other	Professional/ Paraprofessional
1. Loneliness	☐	☐ →	☐	☐	☐	☐
2. Grief/Sadness	☐	☐ →	☐	☐	☐	☐
3. Possible Depression	☐	☐ →	☐	☐	☐	☐
4. Possible Anxiety State	☐	☐ →	☐	☐	☐	☐
5. Verbal Abuse	☐	☐ →	☐	☐	☐	☐
6. Physical Assault Against Others	☐	☐ →	☐	☐	☐	☐
7. Intentional Self Harm	☐	☐ →	☐	☐	☐	☐
8. Verbalizes Suicidal Thoughts/Plans	☐	☐ →	☐	☐	☐	☐
9. Unintentional Self Harm	☐	☐ →	☐	☐	☐	☐
10. Wandering	☐	☐ →	☐	☐	☐	☐
11. Public Disrobing and Public Sexual Behavior	☐	☐ →	☐	☐	☐	☐
12. Probable Undue Suspiciousness of Others	☐	☐ →	☐	☐	☐	☐
13. Probable Hallucinations	☐	☐ →	☐	☐	☐	☐
14. Emotional Instability	☐	☐ →	☐	☐	☐	☐

Comments _____

VIII. ENVIRONMENTAL CONDITIONS

A. Housing Problems ☐ Check, if a licensed health care setting

☐ 1. Air Conditioner
☐ 2. Animals
☐ 3. Building Structure
☐ 4. Cold Water
☐ 5. Dryer
☐ 6. Evaporative Cooler
☐ 7. Freezer Space
☐ 8. Furnishings
☐ 9. Heating
☐ 10. Home Security

☐ 11. Hot Water
☐ 12. Insect/Rodent Infestation
☐ 13. Refrigerator
☐ 14. Stairs
☐ 15. Stove
☐ 16. Telephone
☐ 17. Toilet
☐ 18. Tub/Shower
☐ 19. Washer
☐ 20. Other *(Specify)*

Comments _____

B. Transportation

	Private Transportation		Public Transportation			
	Available		Available		Affordable	
	No	Yes	No	Yes	No	Yes
1. __ To shop for household necessities	☐	☐	☐	☐ →	☐	☐
2. __ To visit family/friends	☐	☐	☐	☐ →	☐	☐
3. __ To obtain medical care	☐	☐	☐	☐ →	☐	☐
4. __ Other *(Specify)*	☐	☐	☐	☐ →	☐	☐

Comments _____

C. Services Being Received Currently (*Check all appropriate boxes*)

☐ 1. None
☐ 2. Adult Day Care
☐ 3. Attendant Care
☐ 4. Chore Maintenance
☐ 5. Counseling
☐ 6. Emergency Notification System Services
☐ 7. Energy Assistance
☐ 8. Errand Services
☐ 9. Escort to Medical
☐ 10. Escort to Other
☐ 11. Financial Budget Assistance
☐ 12. Friendly Visitor
☐ 13. Guardianship/Conservatorship
☐ 14. Home Delivered Meals
☐ 15. Home Health Aid
☐ 16. Home Health Nurse
☐ 17. Home Maintenance
☐ 18. Home Repair
☐ 19. Hospice
☐ 20. Housekeeping
☐ 21. Laundry

☐ 22. Legal Services
☐ 23. Medical Care
☐ 24. Medical Social Services
☐ 25. Nursing Care
☐ 26. Nutrition Services
☐ 27. Occupational Therapy
☐ 28. Ombudsman
☐ 29. Personal Care
☐ 30. Physical Therapy
☐ 31. Protective Services
☐ 32. Public Fiduciary
☐ 33. Recreation/Socialization Services
☐ 34. Respite Sitter
☐ 35. Shopping Service
☐ 36. Speech Therapy
☐ 37. Telephone Reassurance
☐ 38. Transportation
☐ 39. Visiting Nurse
☐ 40. Weatherization
☐ 41. Other *(Specify below)*

Source: Arizona Department of Economic Security, Aging and Adult Administration, 1987.

REFERENCES

American Association of Homes for the Aging. *National Certification Program for Retirement Housing Professionals.* (Rev. ed.) Washington, D.C., 1986.

American Association of Retired Persons (AARP). *A Profile of Older Americans.* Washington, D.C.: AARP, 1985, 1986.

American Health Planning Association. *A Guide for Planning Long Term Care Services for the Elderly.* Washington, D.C., n.d.

Applegate, W. B., and others. "A Geriatric Rehabilitation and Assessment Unit in a Community Hospital." *Journal of the American Geriatrics Society,* 1986, *31* (4), 206–209.

Arizona Department of Economic Security, Aging and Adult Administration. "Arizona Minimum Assessment." Evaluation instrument. Phoenix, Ariz., 1987.

Arizona General Assembly. House of Representatives. Health Committee. *Transcript of the . . . 37th General Assembly, Phoenix, Chapter 199, H. Bill 2029.* Phoenix, Ariz., 1985.

Arnett, R., McKusick, D. R., Sonnefeld, S. T., and Cowell, C. S. "Projections of Healthcare Spending to 1990." *Health Care Financing Review,* 1986, *7* (3), 1–36.

Baker, M. "A Selective Review of Client Assessment Tools in Long Term Care of Older People." Unpublished doctoral dissertation, Florence Heller Graduate School for Advanced Studies in Social Welfare, Brandeis University, 1980.

Blenkner, M. *Protective Services for Older People.* Cleveland: Benjamin Rose Institute, 1974.

Bowersox, J. L. "High Technology and Its Benefits for an Aging Population." Presentation before the U.S. Senate Special Committee on Aging, Washington, D.C., May 22, 1984.

Brickner, P. W. "St. Vincent's Hospital and Medical Center Department of Community Medicine Annual Report." New York: St. Vincent's Hospital, 1985.

Brody, E. M. *Long Term Care of Older People.* New York: Human Science Press, 1977.

Brody, E. M. "Women in the Middle." *The Gerontologist,* 1981, *21,* 471–480.

Brody, E. M. "Parent Care as a Normative Family Stress." *The Gerontologist,* 1985, *25* (1), 19–29.

Brody, S. J., and Magel, J. "Step-Down Care Promotes Vertical Integration." *Hospitals,* 1985, *59* (23), 76–77.

Callahan, J. J., Jr. (ed.). *Major Options in Long-Term Care.* Waltham, Mass.: University Health Policy Consortium, Brandeis University, 1979.

Callahan, J. J., Jr., Diamond, L. D., Giele, J. Z., and Morris, R. "Responsibilities of Families for Their Severely Disabled Elders." *Health Care Financing Review,* 1980, *1* (3), 29–48.

Case Study. Tucson, Ariz.: Pima County Aging and Medical Services Department, Community-Based Programs, n.d.

Cohen, E. S. "Nursing Homes and the Least-Restrictive Environment Doctrine." In M. Kapp, H. Pies, and A. E. Doudera (eds.), *Legal and Ethical Aspects of Health Care.* Ann Arbor, Mich.: Health Administration Press, 1985.

Commonwealth Commission on Elderly Americans Living Alone. *Problems Facing Elderly Americans Living Alone.* New York: Louis Harris and Associates, 1986.

Congressional Clearing House on the Future. *Long Term Care Coverage Gap Threatens Tomorrow's Elderly.* Washington, D.C., 1985a.

Congressional Clearing House on the Future. *Senior Boom: Aging of the U.S. Population Poses Complex Policy Challenge.* Washington, D.C., 1985b.

Doty, P. "Family Care of the Elderly: The Role of Public Policy." *The Milbank Quarterly,* 1986, *64* (1), 34–75.

Drucker, P. F. *Management Tasks, Responsibilities, Practices.* New York: Harper & Row, 1974.

Eisdorfer, C. "Education for Caring." *Bulletin of the New York Academy of Medicine,* 1985, *61* (6), 573–579.

Evashwick, C., Ney, J., and Siemon, J. *Case Management: Issues for Hospitals.* Chicago: Hospital Research and Educational Trust (American Hospital Association), 1985.

Firman, J. "Reforming Community Care for the Elderly and Disabled." *Health Affairs,* 1983, *2* (1), 66–82.

Firshein, J. "Geriatric Evaluation Units Found to Benefit Elderly Patients." *Hospitals,* 1985, *59* (3), 32.

Grauer, H., and Birnbom, F. "A Geriatric Functional Rating Scale to Determine the Need for Institutional Care." *Journal of the American Geriatrics Society,* 1975, *20,* 472–476.

Greenberg, J. N., Leutz, W. N., and Wallack, S. S. "The Social Health Maintenance Organization: A Vertically Integrated Prepaid Care System for the Elderly." *Healthcare Financial Management,* Oct. 1984, pp. 76–86.

Haber, D. "Promoting Mutual Help Groups Among Older People." *The Gerontologist,* 1983, *23* (3), 251–253.

Hodgson, T. A., and Kopstein, A. N. "Health Care Expenditures for Major Diseases in 1980." *Health Care Financing Review,* 1984, *5* (4), 4.

Hughes, S. L. *Long-Term Care Options in an Expanding Market.* Homewood, Ill.: Dow Jones–Irwin, 1986.

Jazwiecki, T. "How to Pay for Long-Term Care Facility Services Under Medicaid." *Healthcare Financial Management,* 1984, *38* (4), 76–78, 80.

Jennings, M. C. "Financing Healthcare Services for the Elderly." In M. T. Kulczycki and M. Peisert (eds.), *The Hospital's Role in Caring for the Elderly: Leadership Issues.* Chicago: Hospital Research and Educational Trust (American Hospital Association), 1982.

Jennings, M. C., and Krentz, S. "Financing Care For the Elderly: Federal Government Programs." In J. Tedesco (ed.),

Financing Quality Care for the Elderly. Chicago: Hospital Research and Educational Trust (American Hospital Association), 1985.

Kane, R. A., and Kane, R. L. *Assessing the Elderly.* Lexington, Mass.: Heath, 1981.

Katz, S., and Akpom, A. "A Measure of Primary Biological and Social Functioning." *International Journal of Health Services,* 1976, *6* (3), 494.

Katzper, M. *Modeling of Long Term Care.* Human Services Monograph Series, no. 21. Washington, D.C.: Department of Health and Human Services, 1981.

Koch, K. *I Never Told Anybody: Teaching Poetry Writing in a Nursing Home.* New York: Random House, 1977.

Koff, T. H. *Long-Term Care: An Approach to Serving the Frail Elderly.* Boston: Little, Brown, 1982.

Kovar, M. G. "Aging in the Eighties." In *Vital and Health Statistics of the National Center for Health Statistics.* Washington, D.C.: Department of Health and Human Services, 1986.

Laventhal and Horwath. "Lifecare Retirement Center Industry Annual Report." Philadelphia: Laventhal and Horwath, 1985.

Lawton, M. P. "Social Ecology and the Health of Older People." *American Journal of Public Health,* 1974, *64* (3), 257–260.

Lawton, M. P. "Assessing the Competence of Older People." In D. P. Kent and others (eds.), *Research, Planning, and Action for the Elderly.* New York: Behavioral Publications, 1976.

Leanse, J., Tiven, M., and Robb, T. B. *Senior Center Operation.* Washington, D.C.: National Council on Aging, 1977.

Leutz, W. N., and others. *Changing Health Care for an Aging Society.* Lexington, Mass.: Heath, 1985.

Liu, K., Manton, K. G., and Liu, B. "Home Care for the Disabled Elderly." *Health Care Financing Review,* 1985, *7* (2), 51–58.

Lubkin, I. M. *Chronic Illness: Impact and Interventions.* Boston: Jones and Bartlett, 1986.

Maddox, G. (ed.). *The Encyclopedia of Aging.* New York: Springer, 1987.

Mayo, C. "Problems and Challenges." In *Guide to Action on Chronic Illness.* New York: National Health Council, 1956.

Meiners, M. R., and Gollub, J. O. "Long-Term Care Insurance: The Edge of the Emerging Market." *Caring,* Mar. 1985, pp. 12–16.

Miller, D. B. "Societal Changes and the Human Resource Component in Long Term Care." In *Proceedings of the Second National Conference on Long Term Care Issues.* Tacoma, Wash.: Hillhaven Foundation, 1982.

Moore, J., and others. "Evolution of a Geriatric Evaluation Clinic." *Journal of the American Geriatrics Society,* 1984, *32* (12), 900–905.

Morris, J. N., Sherwood, S., and Mor, V. "An Assessment Tool for Use in Identifying Functionally Vulnerable Persons in the Community." *The Gerontologist,* 1984, *24* (4), 373–379.

Mt. Zion Hospital and Medical Center. (Handout). San Francisco: Mt. Zion Hospital and Medical Center, n.d.

National Center for Health Statistics. *National Nursing Home Survey: 1977—Summary for the United States.* DHEW Publication no. (PHS) 79-1794. Vital and Health Statistics Series 13, no. 43. Hyattsville, Md.: National Center for Health Statistics, July 1979.

National Long Term Care Survey 1982 and National Survey of Informal Caregivers 1982. Washington, D.C.: Department of Health and Human Services, 1982.

Nelson, L. S. "The Law, Professional Responsibility, and Decisions to Forego Treatment." *QRB,* Jan. 1986, pp. 8–15.

Nursing Homes: All About Them; How to Pick One. Rochester, Minn.: Mayo Clinic, 1987.

Older Americans Act of 1965 (Public Law 89-73).

Olson, E., Prochnow, J., and Zalenko, M. "Hospital-Based Case Management Coordination." *Continuing Care Coordinator,* 1986, *5* (4), 20–22.

Park Plaza Retirement Residences. Cost analysis form. Orange, Calif., 1987.

Phillips, L. R., and Rempusheski, V. F. "Making Decisions About Elder Abuse." *Social Casework: The Journal of Contemporary Social Work,* Mar. 1986, pp. 131–140.

Profile (brochure). San Francisco: On Lok Senior Health Services, n.d.

Raschko, B. B. *Housing Interiors for the Disabled and Elderly.* New York: Van Nostrand Reinhold, 1982.

Reidel, R. L. *Long Term Care Systems for the Elderly.* Chicago:

Hospital Research and Educational Trust (American Hospital Association), 1984.

Rice, J. A., and Taylor, S. "Assess the Market for Long Term Care Service." *Healthcare Financial Management,* Feb. 1984, pp. 35–46.

Rubenstein, L. Z. "The Clinical Effectiveness of Multidimensional Geriatric Assessment." *Journal of the American Geriatrics Society,* 1983, *31* (12), 758–762.

Rubenstein, L. Z. "Geriatric Imperatives: Geriatric Assessment Programs." *Journal of the Medical Society of New Jersey,* 1984, *81* (8), 651–654.

Rubenstein, L. Z., Rhee, L., and Kane, R. L. "The Role of Geriatric Assessment Units in Caring for the Elderly: An Analysis Review." *Journal of Gerontology,* 1982, *37* (5), 513–521.

Scanlon, W. J., and Feder, J. "The Long-Term Marketplace: An Overview." *Healthcare Financial Management,* 1984, *14* (3), 42–44, 48, 50, 52, 54.

Schiffer, C. F. "DNR Doesn't Stand for 'Do Not Respect.'" *Medical Economics,* Feb. 1987, pp. 29–32.

Schorr, A. L. *"Thy Father and Thy Mother . . . ": A Second Look at Filial Responsibility and Family Policy.* Washington, D.C.: Department of Health and Human Services, 1980.

Shore, H. "Surviving as an Administrator." *Contemporary Long Term Care,* 1987, *10* (10), 38–42.

Siu, A. L., Brook, R. P., and Rubenstein, L. Z. "Medicare Capitation and Quality of Care for the Frail Elderly." *Health Care Financing Review,* 1986 Annual Supplement, pp. 57–61.

Soldo, B. "The Elderly Home Care Population: National Prevalence Rates, Select Characteristics, and Alternative Sources of Assistance." In *Project to Analyze Existing Long Term Care Data: Final Report.* Vol. 3. Washington, D.C.: Department of Health and Human Services, 1983.

Somers, A. R. "Financing Long-Term Care for the Elderly: Institutions, Incentives, Issues." In *America's Aging Health in an Older Society.* Washington, D.C.: National Academy Press, 1985.

A Step Toward Independence. Milwaukee, Wisc.: Sinai Samaritan Medical Center, Oct. 1985.

Stephens, S. A., and Christianson, J. B. *Informal Care of the Elderly*. Lexington, Mass.: Heath, 1986.

Stone, R. "Aging in the Eighties: Age 65 Years and Over—Use of Community Services." In *Vital and Health Statistics of the National Center for Health Statistics*. Washington, D.C.: Department of Health and Human Services, 1986.

Stone, R., Cafferata, G. L., and Sangl, J. "Caregiving the Frail Elderly: A National Profile." *The Gerontologist*, 1987, *27* (5), 616–626.

Strauss, A. L., and others. *Chronic Illness and the Quality of Life*. St. Louis, Mo.: Mosby, 1984.

Thomasma, D. C. "Freedom, Dependency, and the Care of the Very Old." *Journal of the American Geriatrics Society*, 1984, *32* (12), 906–914.

Torrey, B. B., Kinsella, K. G., and Taeuber, C. M. *An Aging World*. Advance report to the U.S. Bureau of the Census. Washington, D.C., 1987.

Tymchuk, A. J., Auslander, J. G., and Rader, N. "Informing the Elderly: A Comparison of Four Methods." *Journal of the American Geriatrics Society*, 1986, *34*, 818–822.

U.S. Bureau of the Census. *Population Estimates and Projections*. Series P-25, no. 937. Washington, D.C., 1983.

U.S. General Accounting Office. *Entering a Nursing Home: Costly Implications for Medicaid and the Elderly*. Washington, D.C., 1979.

U.S. Senate Special Committee on Aging. *Developments in Aging: 1986*. Vol. 1. Washington, D.C., 1987.

U.S. Senate Special Committee on Aging, in conjunction with the American Association of Retired Persons, the Federal Council on Aging, and the Administration on Aging. *Aging America: Trends and Projections*. (1985 and 1986 eds.) Washington, D.C., 1985, 1986.

Valiente, J. D. "The Capital Requirements for Long Term Care Services." *Healthcare Financial Management*, Apr. 1984, pp. 84–90.

Waldo, D., Levit, K., and Lazenby, H. "National Health Expenditures." *Health Care Financing Review*, 1986, *8* (1), 1–21.

Warren, J. W., and others. "Informed Consent by Proxy." *New England Journal of Medicine*, 1986, *315* (18), 1124–1156.

Wetle, T. T. "Ethical Aspects of Decision Making for and with the Elderly." In M. B. Kapp and others (eds.), *Legal and*

Ethical Aspects of Health Care for the Elderly. Ann Arbor, Mich.: Health Administration Press, 1985.

Wright, B. A. *Physical Disability: A Psychological Approach*. New York: Harper & Row, 1960.

Young, L., Harnett, E. R., Brickner, P. W., and Scharer, L. K. *Annual Report 1985*. New York: St. Vincent's Hospital and Medical Center of New York, 1985.

INDEX

A

AARP Andrus Foundation, 212

ABC Chronic Care Program, planning by, 106

Abuse, of elderly, 200–202

Accreditation Council for Development of Services for Mentally Retarded and Other Developmentally Disabled Persons, 218

Administration on Aging, 79, 126, 153

Adult day health care: design criteria for, 148; implementation plan for, 154; settings for, 47–49

Adult Protective Services (APS), 24, 28

Advocacy: and care coordination, 179; and counseling, 39–40

Aid to Families with Dependent Children, 230

AIDS, and new programs, 166

Akpom, A., 168

Albuquerque, hospital chronic care in, 67

Alzheimer's disease: adult day health services for, 48; family support group for, 78–79, 126; geriatric services for, 87; and new programs, 166

Alzheimer's Disease and Related Disorders Association (ADRDA), 78–79, 224

American Association for Continuity of Care, 214–215

American Association of Homes for the Aging, 59, 158, 160, 220–221

American Association of Retired Persons (AARP), 1, 3*n*, 6, 7*n*, 73, 211–212

American Coalition of Citizens with Disabilities, 212

American College of Health Care Administrators, 221

American College of Healthcare Executives, 158, 217

American Dietetic Association, 222

American Federation of Home Health Agencies, 215

American Geriatrics Society, 159, 212–213

American Health Care Association, 158, 160, 221
American Health Planning Association, 31
American Hospital Association, 158, 161, 216–217
American Medical Association, 158
American Medical Directors Association, 221–222
American Nurses' Association, 158, 219
American Protestant Health Association, 224
American Society for Parenteral and Enteral Nutrition, 222
American Society on Aging, 159, 160, 213
Applegate, W. B., 168
Area Agency on Aging, 40, 106–107, 126, 153–155, 156, 162, 209, 211
Arizona: AHCCS program in, 47; assessment in, 233–249. See also Pima and Tucson entries
Arizona, University of, College of Nursing at, 43
Arizona Association of Nonprofit Nursing Homes, 160
Arizona Bureau of Aging, 44
Arizona Department of Economic Security, Aging and Adult Administration, 44, 249n
Arizona General Assembly, 205n
Arizona Long Term Care Gerontology Center, 79
Armory Park Senior Center: nutrition site at, 44, 45; services of, 42–43
Arts, in services for elderly, 49–50
Assessment: benefits of, 167–168; and care coordinator, 170; of clients, 167–176; criteria for, 175; for family members, 169; of functional capacities, 168; instruments for, 171–174, 233–249
Association for Retarded Citizens, 218
Association of Western Hospitals, 161
Auslander, J. G., 203

B

Baker, M., 169, 170
Birnbom, F., 170, 172n, 173

Blenkner, M. 73
Blue Cross/Blue Shield, and licensed home health care, 46
Bowersox, J. L., 132
Brandeis University, Health Policy Center at, 123–124, 209
Brethren Homes for the Aged, 224
Brickner, P. W., 32
Brody, E. M., 17, 18, 71, 76
Brody, S. J., 68
Brookdale Foundation, 43
Brookhurst Hospital, planning by, 99
Brooklyn, social HMO in, 34, 124, 125

C

Cafferata, G. L., 76
California: congregate housing in, 61; demonstration project in, 34; social HMO in, 34, 124, 125. See also Mount Zion and On Lok programs
California Acute Rehabilitation, 162
California Adult Day Care, 162
California Adult Day Health Center, 161
California Association for Health Services at Home, 160
California Association of Adult Day Care Centers, 161
California Association of Adult Day Services, 160
California Association of Home Health Agencies, 161
California Association of Homes for the Aging, 160
California Community Clinic, 161
California Department of Health Services, 82
California Health Care Service Plan, 161
California Home Health Agency, 161
California Home Health Care, 162
California Hospital, 162
California Skilled Nursing Care, 162
Callahan, J. J., Jr., 71–72, 177
Care coordination: and advocacy, 179; case studies of, 180–181; concept of, 19, 176–177; existing, 179–180; operation of, 178–179; program for, 176–181; results of, 177–178

Case management. *See* Care coordination

Catholic Community Services, 44

Catholic Health Association of the United States, 217

Channeling Demonstration Projects, 34, 75

Chelsea-Village Program (CVP), long-term care in, 83–84

Christianson, J. B., 75

Chronic care services: administration of, 165–210; brokered approach to, 69, 167; case studies of, 42–43, 44–45, 46–47, 48–49; and chronic illness, 16–35; circular design of, 53–54; community service model for, 56–57; complexity of, 20–27; concept of, 19, 21; congregate housing and services models of, 57–62; constituencies for, 182–195; coordinated, 27–29, 81–90; delivery of, 81–164; demand for, 1–15; demonstration programs in, 34; designing, 52–56; designing environments for, 129–149; determining appropriate, 26–27; for disabled, 24–25; family role in, 71–80; federated approach to, 69–70; financing, 110–128; formats for delivery of, 68–70; foundations for success of, 208–210; future of, 13–15; guidelines for, 209–210; home care model of, 63–65; implementing, 150–164; importance of, 22; institutional care model for, 65–68; insurance coverage for, 227–231; linear design of, 53; management of, 182–183; models of, 56–68, 81–90; network for, 185; operation of programs for, 165–181; organizations for, 211–226; organizing and delivering, 52–70; paying for, 117–128; personal rights in, 196–207; philosophy and goal statement for, 29–33; planning, 91–109; providing, 1–80; sponsorship and components of, 33–35; terminology in, 18–19; types of, 36–51; vertical integration of, 68–69, 108–109

Chronic illness: analysis of responding to, 16–35; case studies of, 22–25, 26–27, 28–29; complexity of, 20–27; concept of, 25; considerations in, 20–21; continuum used in, 28–29; long-term care for, 17–18; trajectory of, 20

Church of the Brethren Homes and Hospital, 224–25

Cohen, E. S., 196

Columbia University, 50

Community, as constituency, 187–188

Community groups, and implementation, 162–164

Community resources: and planning, 98–99; utilization of, 12–13

Community service model, organization of, 56–57

Congregate housing: concept of, 57; design criteria for, 147–148; organization of, 57–62

Congressional Clearing House on the Future, 14

Consent: for research, 206; and rights, 203–206

Constituencies: analysis of interacting with, 182–195; background on, 182–184; community as, 187–188; elderly as, 188–189; family as, 189–190; owners as, 188; physicians as, 190–191; public officials as, 184–186; staff as, 192–195; volunteers as, 191–192

Costs, types of, 151–153

Counseling, service of, 38–40

D

Decision not to resuscitate (DNR), and ethics committees, 204–206

Delivery models, case studies of, 56–57, 61–62, 82–90

Department of Community Medicine, and long-term care, 83, 84

Design: analysis of, 129–149; background on, 129–131; criteria for, 131, 132–136; and family needs, 149; of nursing homes, 137–147; of personal-care facility, 142; for specialized programs, 136–148; and staff needs, 148–149

Diagnosis-related groups (DRGs): and

coordinated programs, 34; and hospital chronic care, 67; and licensed home health care, 46
Diamond, L. D., 72
Division of Ambulatory Care, 217
Doty, P., 72, 80
Downtown Hospital, planning by, 105
Drucker, P. F., 182

E

Ebenezer Society, and social HMO, 124, 125
Eisdorfer, C., 91
Elderly: abuse of, 200–202; assessment of, 167–176; associations of, 211–212; background on, 1–5; bill of rights for, 199–200; chronic illness for, 16–35; community groups of, 162–164; community services used by, 12–13; concept of, 19; consequences of growing population of, 5–13; as constituency, 188–189; and demand for services, 1–15; designing environments for, 129–149; designing services for, 52–56; facts about, 1–3; and health care expenditures, 9; impairment/disability/handicap for, 26; implications for, 14–15; independence for, 23–24; personal rights of, 196–207; and population trends, 4; rehabilitation needs of, 10–11; services for, 36–51; trends for, 14
Elderplan, as social HMO, 124, 125
Environmental press, and design criteria, 145. *See also* Design
Ethics committees, and decision not to resuscitate, 204–206. *See also* Rights
Evashwick, C., 33–34, 177

F

Family: assessment for, 169; case study of, 79–80; chronic care role of, 71–80; as constituency, 189–190; designing for needs of, 149; education for, 206–207; and filial responsibility, 73; magnitude of care by, 76–78; peer support groups for, 78–79; policy changes for, 80
Federal Housing Administration (FHA), 117
Federation of Southern Arizona, 44
Financing: analysis of, 110–128; background on, 110–111; capital, 116–117; and expanded service role, 111–115; federal programs for, 118; from grants, 127; and implementation, 151–153; and integration of services, 115–116; market assessment for, 111; and paying for chronic care, 117–128; and planning, 98; public sources of, 120–121; from waivers, 127–128
Firman, J., 13
Firshein, J., 11
Foster care, organization of, 61

G

Geriatric Functional Rating Scale, 170–172
Geriatrics Institute, services of, 87, 89
Gerontological Society of America, 159, 213
Gerontology and geriatrics, associations for, 212–214
Giele, J. Z., 72
Glenborough Hospital, planning by, 95–96
Gollub, J. O., 123
Grauer, H., 170, 172n, 173
Greenberg, J. N., 123, 124, 125n
Group Health, Inc., and social HMO, 124
Group homes, organization of, 60–61

H

H & R Block, 47
Haber, D., 78
Handmaker Jewish Geriatric Center: adult day health services at, 48–49, 90; nutrition site at, 44
Harnett, E. R., 32
Health Care Financing Administration, 74, 215

Health Insurance Association of America, 231

Health maintenance organizations (HMOs): and care coordination, 179, 180; co-opting by, 105; and coordinated services, 35; financing, 122; and home care, 64; and integrated services, 156. *See also* Social HMOs

Hearing, and design criteria, 132-133

Hebrew Rehabilitation Center for the Aged, assessment by, 173

Hodgson, T. A., 9n

Home care: associations for, 214-216; services of, 63-65

Home health services: benefits of, 55-56; categories of, 45-47

Home Health Services and Staffing Association, 215

Homemaker services, and home health care, 47

Horwath, 60

Hospice care: association for, 216; services of, 50-51

Hospital Initiatives in Long-Term Care, 34, 87

Hospitals: administration of, associations for, 216-217; chronic care in, 66-67; and nursing care unit design, 143, 145-146; potential services of, 112-115; teaching, and joint venture, 107

HRCA Vulnerability Index, 173-174

Hughes, S. L., 52, 110, 150

I

Implementation: analysis of, 150-164; and Area Agency on Aging, 153-155; case studies of, 152, 163; and community groups, 162-164; costs in, 151-153; and integrated medical and social services, 156-157; and licensing, 161-162; plan for, 153-154; and staff orientation, 157-161

Institutional care model, organization of, 65-68

Insurance: coverage summaries for, 227-231; for long-term care, 231; private, and chronic care financing, 123-124

Intermediate care, concept of, 65-66

J

Jawiecki, T., 122

Jennings, M. C., 116, 121n

Joint venture, and planning, 105-108

K

Kaiser Permanente Medical Care Program, as social HMO, 124, 125

Kane, R. A., 165, 169, 172, 173, 174, 175n, 177

Kane, R. L., 165, 168, 169, 172, 173, 174, 175n

Katz, S., 168

Katzper, M., 81

Kellogg Foundation, 43

Kinsella, K. G., 1

Koch, K., 50

Koff, T. H., 17

Kopstein, A. N., 9n

Kovar, M. G., 12

Krentz, S., 121n

L

Laventhal, 60

Law, associations on, 217-218

Lawton, M. P., 145, 170

Leanse, J., 40

Leutz, W. N., 116, 123, 124, 125n

Licensed home health care, services of, 45-47

Licensing, and implementation, 161-162

Life Care at Home Program, 124, 209

Lifecare Retirement Center Industry, 60

Liu, B., 72

Liu, K., 72

Living Will, and rights, 205-206

Lombardi Law (New York), 63

Long Beach, social HMO in, 34, 124, 125

Long-term care, defining, 17-18

Long Term Care Survey, 74, 76
Lubkin, I. M., 20, 36

M

Maddox, G., 37
Magel, J., 68
Manton, K. G., 72
Market: assessment of, 111; and competitive position, 102–103; evaluation of, for planning, 99–103; survey report on, 103; target segments of, 100–102
Mayo, C., 16
Medicaid: alternative to, 47; benefits from, 8, 14, 84, 111, 122–123, 208; and bill of rights, 199; capitation financing from, 83; coverage by, 227, 229–230; and demonstration projects, 34; and informal providers, 73; and institutional care guidelines, 65; and licensing, 162; and 1115 waivers, 83, 127; passage of, 16; and payment relationships, 183; and preadmission screening, 11; and 2176 waivers, 230
Medical Personnel Pool, and licensed home health care, 45–47
Medicare: benefits from, 8, 34, 111, 119, 122, 123, 208; and bill of rights, 199; capitation financing from, 83; coverage by, 227, 228–229; and demonstration projects, 34; and hospice care, 51; and informal providers, 73; and institutional care guidelines, 65; issues of, 215; and licensed home health care, 46; passage of, 16; and payment relationships, 183; and supplemental insurance, 85–86, 231; support for, 212; and 222 waivers, 83, 127
Medicare Partners, as social HMO, 124, 125
Medicare Plus II, as social HMO, 125
Medigap, coverage by, 230–231
Meiners, M. R., 123
Mental Health and retardation, associations on, 218–219
Mental Retardation Association of America, 218

Metropolitan Jewish Geriatric Center, social HMO of, 124, 125
Midtown Nursing Home, planning by, 108
Miller, D. B., 129
Milwaukee. *See* Sinai Samaritan program
Minimum Assessment Instrument, 233–249
Minneapolis: and design criteria, 132; social HMO in, 34, 124
Mission, in planning, 93–94, 104–105
Mission Plaza Retirement Community, and start-up costs, 152
Mobility and agility, and design criteria, 135–136
Model Cities project, 44
Moore, J., 168
Mor, V., 174n
Morris, J. N., 174n
Morris, R., 72
Mount Zion Care Account, 85–86
Mt. Zion Hospital and Medical Center: affiliations of, 161; arts at, 49; described, 84–86; goal of, 32–33; licenses of, 162; success of, 209
Multipurpose Senior Services Project, 34

N

National Alliance for the Mentally Ill, 219
National Association for Home Care, 158, 215
National Association for Senior Living Industries, 158
National Association of Area Agencies on Aging, 211
National Association of Meal Programs, 223
National Association of Nutrition and Aging, 223
National Association of Social Workers, 223
National Caucus and Center on Black Aged, 225
National Center for Health Statistics, 11
National Center on Rural Aging, 213–214

National Channelling Demonstration Program, 75

National Council of Senior Citizens, 212

National Council on Aging, 158, 159, 160, 213–214

National Federation of Licensed Practical Nurses, 219–220

National Fire Protection Association Life Safety Code, 147

National Foundation for Long Term Health Care, 222

National Hispanic Council on Aging, 225

National Homecaring Council, 216

National Hospice Organization, 158, 216

National Indian Council on Aging, 225

National Institute of Senior Centers, 214

National Institute of Senior Housing, 214

National Institute on Adult Day Care, 160, 214

National Institute on Community-Based Long-Term Care, 214

National League for Nursing, 220

National Long-Term Care Survey, 76

National Mental Health Association, 219

National Pacific/Asian Resource Center on Aging, 226

National Retired Teachers Association, 212

National Senior Citizens Education and Research Center, 212

National Senior Citizens Law Center, 217–218

National Training Center on Aging, 213

National Voluntary Organizations for Independent Living for the Aging, 214

Neighborhood-based caregiver network, and family support, 79–80

Nelson, L. S., 204

New Mexico, hospital chronic care in, 67

New York: demonstration project in, 34; home care law in, 63; nursing home without walls program in, 84.

See also St. Vincent's Hospital and Medical Center of New York

New York Hospital, 162

New York Long Term Home Care, 162

New York Short Term Home Care, 162

Ney, J., 33–34, 177

North American Association of Jewish Homes and Housing for the Aged, 226

Nursing, associations for, 219–220

Nursing Home Without Walls, 34, 64, 84

Nursing homes: associations for, 220–222; categories of care in, 65–66; circular design of, 139–140; code conformity for, 146–147; design of, 137–147; modular design for, 144; site selection for, 146; typical design of, 138

Nutrition: associations for, 222–223; services for, 43–45

O

Office of Human Development, 126

Older Americans Act of 1965, 16, 40, 43, 48, 111, 126, 153, 154, 164, 179. *See also* Title III

Olson, E., 89

Omnibus Budget Reconciliation Act (OBRA) of 1981, 34

On Lok Senior Health Services: affiliations of, 160; described, 82–83; financing, 122, 123, 127; goal of, 32; licenses of, 161; success of, 208; vertical integration of, 109

Orange, California, congregate housing in, 61

Oregon, social HMO in, 34, 124, 125

Orientation: and design criteria, 133–134, 141, 145; of staff, 157–161, 193–194

Owners, as constituency, 188

P

Park Plaza Retirement Residences, and congregate housing, 61–62

Pascua Indian Center, nutrition site at, 45

Paternalism, and rights, 197–198

Personal-care services: concept of, 66; designing for, 142; and home health care, 47

Personalization, and design criteria, 134–135

Personnel Pool of America, 47

Phillips, L. R., 200

Physicians, as constituency, 190–191

Pima Council on Aging, 43, 44, 209

Pima County: funding by, 90; licensed home health care in, 45–47

Pima County Aging and Medical Services: affiliations of, 160; described, 89–90; family support program of, 79; and financing, 126; goal of, 32; license of, 161–162; success of, 209

Pima County Long Term Care System, and coordination, 155

Pima County Nutrition Sites, services of, 44–45

Planning: alternatives assessed in, 103–109; analysis of, 91–109; background on, 91–92; case studies of, 95–97, 99, 105, 106–107, 108; and community resources, 98–99; and co-opting services, 105; costs of, 151; and financing, 98; for future direction, 92–94; and implementation, 153–154; and internal resources, 94–97; and joint venture, 105–108; and market evaluation, 99–103; mission in, 93–94, 104–105; and obstacles, 98; and philosophy, 92–93; strategies in, 94–99; for vertical integration, 108–109

Portland, Oregon, social HMO in, 34, 124, 125

Posada del Sol Nursing Home, services of, 89, 90

Preferred provider organization (PPO), at Mount Zion, 86

Presbyterian Health Care, 67

Prochnow, J., 89

Program for Hospital Initiatives for Long-Term Care, 87

Programs: analysis of operating, 165–181; assessment in, 167–176; background on, 165–166; for care coordination, 176–181; controlled access to, 166–167

Project Age Well, 43

Providers, formal and informal, 72

Psychiatric Day Care, 162.

Public Law 89-73. See Older Americans Act

Public officials, as constituency, 184–186

Q

Quality of life, and rights, 202–203

R

Rader, N., 203

Raschko, B. B., 131

Rehabilitation: need for, 10–11; service of, 36–38

Rempusheski, V. F., 200

Research, consent for, 206

Respite care, services of, 50

Reverse Mortgage Program, 29

Rhee, L., 168

Rice, J. A., 111, 112

Rights: analysis of protecting, 196–207; background on, 196–197; bill of, 199–200; and consent, 203–206; and education of staff and family, 206–207; and elder abuse, 200–202; and paternalism, 197–198; and quality of life, 202–203

Riverview Manors, planning by, 96–97

Robb, T. B., 40

Robert Wood Johnson Foundation, 34, 64, 87, 124, 208

Rubenstein, L. Z., 167, 168

S

St. Vincent's Hospital and Medical Center of New York: affiliations of, 161; described, 83–84; goal of, 32; home care program of, 64; integrated services of, 156–157; licenses of, 162; success of, 209

Salvation Army, 44

San Francisco. See Mount Zion and On Lok programs

San Francisco Institute on Aging, 33, 84–85, 86, 161, 162

Sangl, J., 76
SCAN Health Plan, as social HMO, 124, 125
Scharer, L. K., 32
Schiffer, C. F., 204
Schorr, A. L., 73
Section 8, 24, 90
Section 202/8, 127, 161
Section 222, 34, 83, 127
Section 1115, 34, 83, 127
Section 2176, 34
Senior Care Action Network, social HMO of, 124, 125
Senior centers, services of, 40–43
Senior Now Generation, 44
Sherwood, S., 174n
Shore, H., 208
Siemon, J., 33–34, 177
Sinai Samaritan Medical Center: described, 87–89; goal of, 32; success of, 209
Skilled care, concept of, 65
Social health maintenance organizations (S/HMOs): demonstration projects for, 34, 125; development of, 209; financing, 123–124; and home care, 64; at hospitals, 113–114; and waivers, 127
Social Security, 212; Amendments of 1983 for, 4. See also Title XX
Social Services Block Grants, 90, 111, 124, 126; Title XX funds, 45
Social work, associations on, 223–224
Society for Hospital Social Work Directors, 224
Soldo, B., 72
Somers, A. R., 119
South Park Area Council Center, 44
Southside Hospital, planning by, 106–107
Special Constituency Section of Aging and Long Term Care, 217
Spiritual supports, provision of, 49
Staff: compensation for, 194–195; as constituency, 192–195; designing for needs of, 148–149; education for, 206–207; and elder abuse, 202; orientation of, 157–161, 193–194; and paternalism, 198; trade or professional associations for, 157–159

Stephens, S. A., 75
Stone, R., 12, 13n, 76
Strauss, A. L., 21
Sunrise Health Care Corporation, planning by, 108
Supplemental Security Income (SSI), 80, 230

T

Taeuber, C. M., 1
Tax Equity and Fiscal Responsibility Act (TEFRA) of 1982, 34
Taylor, S., 111, 112
Thomasma, D. C., 197
Title III of Older Americans Act, 43, 44, 45, 46, 90, 117
Title VII of Older Americans Act, 44
Title 19, 90
Title XX, 24, 28, 45, 49, 90, 179
Tiven, M., 40
Torrey, B. B., 1
Touch, and design criteria, 133
Transportation, services for, 43
Tucson, Arizona: adult day health services in, 48–49; chronic care in, 184; nutrition sites in, 44–45; senior center in, 42–43. See also Pima entries
Tucson Jewish Community Center, and nutrition sites, 44
Tucson Medical Center, and chronic care, 184
Tucson Metropolitan Ministries, 44
Tymchuck, A. J., 203

U

U.S. Bureau of the Census, 4n
U.S. Department of Health and Human Services, 14, 17, 18, 153, 230
U.S. Department of Housing and Urban Development (HUD), 58, 11, 127, 161; and Section 8 funds, 24, 90
U.S. General Accounting Office, 118n
U.S. Senate Special Committee on Aging, 74, 227
United Way, 45, 49, 90

V

Valiente, J. D., 5, 11
Veterans Administration, 111, 126–127
Vision, design criteria for, 132
Visiting Nurse Associations of America, 220
Volunteers, as constituency, 191–192

W

Wallack, S. S., 123, 124n, 125
Warren, J. W., 206

Western Gerontological Society, 213
Westwood Retirement Community, and community groups, 163
Wetle, T. T., 198
Wisconsin. *See* Sinai Samaritan program

Y

Young, L., 32

Z

Zalenko, M., 89

The case studies in Chapter Three are included herein with the approval of Armory Park Senior Citizens Center, Tucson, Ariz.; Pima County Council on Aging, Tucson, Ariz.; Medical Personnel Pool, Tucson, Ariz.; and Handmaker Jewish Geriatric Center, Tucson, Ariz.

The case studies in Chapter Six are included herein with the approval of On Lok Senior Health Services, San Francisco, Calif.; St. Vincent's Hospital and Medical Center of New York, New York, N.Y.; Mt. Zion Health Systems, Inc., San Francisco, Calif.; Sinai Samaritan Medical Center, Milwaukee, Wisc.; and Department of Aging and Medical Services, Tucson, Ariz.